Doctoral Education in Nursing

International Perspectives

Over the last one hundred years the nursing role has evolved to become a high-profile professional discipline in which evidence-based practice has become increasingly important both for nurses and for their patients. More recently, this has resulted in a large increase in the number of nurses wishing to broaden their knowledge base and to study for doctorates. Until now, however, there has been no text specifically related to doctoral education in the nursing or midwifery context – *Doctoral Education in Nursing*: *International Perspectives* fills that gap.

This book takes a truly international approach to examining best practice in doctoral education, covering the following topics:

- what doctoral study in nursing involves
- the roles of the student, the supervisor, the awarding institution
- the doctoral process
- quality indicators
- funding
- models of international exchange
- postdoctoral study

This book will rapidly become an indispensable source of reference for doctoral students and their mentors, wherever they are pursuing their research.

Shaké Ketefian is Professor and Director of International Affairs at the University of Michigan School of Nursing. She has published widely in ethical practice and ethical decision making, and on doctoral education, within the USA and internationally. She served as the director of doctoral and postdoctoral programmes at her institution for 17 years, and is currently the President of the International Network for Doctoral Education in Nursing. She is the recipient of a number of awards. Dr Ketefian is also the Editor of *Research and Theory for Nursing Practice: An International Journal.*

Hugh P. McKenna is Head of the School of Nursing at the University of Ulster. He has published widely on doctoral education in nursing. He is also Treasurer of the International Network for Doctoral Education in Nursing and has been awarded a number of international honours including a Fellowship of the European Academy of Nursing Science and a Fellowship of the Royal College of Nursing.

This book is dedicated to the International Network for Doctoral Education in Nursing and its members. The support and commitment of the members to achieving excellence in international doctoral education inspired and made this book a reality.

Doctoral Education in Nursing

International Perspectives

Shaké Ketefian and Hugh P. McKenna

Routledge
Taylor & Francis Group
LONDON AND NEW YORK

First published in 2005 by Routledge
2 Park Square, Milton Park, Abingdon, Oxon OX14 4RN

Simultaneously published in the USA and Canada
by Routledge
29 West 35th Street, New York, NY 10001

Routledge is an imprint of the Taylor & Francis Group

Typeset in Sabon MT by J&L Composition, Filey, North Yorkshire
Printed and bound in Great Britain by The Cromwell Press, Trowbridge

British Library Cataloguing in Publication Data
A catalogue record for this book is available from the British Library

Library of Congress Cataloging in Publication Data
A catalogue record has been requested

ISBN 0 415 31900 5 (Pbk)
ISBN 0 415 31899 8 (Hbk)

Contents

Contributors

Lynn Chenoweth, PhD, RN
Professor of Aged and Extended Care Nursing; and Director
Faculty of Nursing, Midwifery and Health
University of Technology, Sydney, Australia

Mary Courtney, PhD, RN
Director of Research, School of Nursing
Queensland University of Technology, Australia

John R. Cutcliffe, PhD, RN
Chair of Nursing
University of Northern British Columbia, Canada

Dawn Freshwater, PhD, RN
Professor of Mental Health and Primary Care
Bournemouth University, UK

Kate Galvin, PhD, RN
Professor and Head of Research Institute of Health and Community Studies
Bournemouth University, UK

Morag A. Gray, PhD, MN, RGN, I.L.T.M.
Head of Curriculum Development; Reader and Senior Teaching Fellow
Faculty of Health and Life Sciences
Napier University, Edinburgh, UK

Somchit Hanucharurnkul, PhD, RN
Professor and Director of the Doctoral Program
Ramathibodi School of Nursing, Bangkok, Thailand

Ada Sue Hinshaw, PhD, RN, FAAN
Professor and Dean, School of Nursing
University of Michigan, Ann Arbor, MI, USA

Shaké Ketefian, EdD, RN, FAAN
Professor and Director of International Affairs, School of Nursing
University of Michigan, Ann Arbor, MI, USA

Mi Ja Kim, PhD, RN, FAAN
Professor and Dean Emeritus
Director, Academy of International Leadership Development
University of Illinois at Chicago, IL, USA

Eun-Ok Lee, PhD, RN
Professor, College of Nursing
Seoul National University, Korea

Helena Leino-Kilpi, PhD, RN
Professor; Head of the Department of Nursing Science
University of Turku, Finland

Carol Loveland-Cherry, PhD, RN, FAAN
Professor and Executive Associate Dean, Academic Affairs
Interim Director, Doctoral and Postgraduate Studies
University of Michigan, Ann Arbor, MI, USA

Hugh P. McKenna, PhD, RN
Professor and Dean, School of Nursing
University of Ulster at Jordantown, UK

Afaf I. Meleis PhD, RN, Dr PS (hon), FAAN, Dean
Professor of Nursing and Sociology; and Dean
University of Pennsylvania School of Nursing, USA

Kristen S. Montgomery, PhD, RN
Assistant Professor, College of Nursing
University of South Carolina, Columbia, USA

Jody D. Nyquist, PhD
Associate Dean Emeritus, The Graduate School
Former Director, The Re-envisioning the PhD Project
University of Washington, Seattle, USA

Joanne Olson, PhD, RN
Professor and Assistant Dean, Faculty of Nursing
University of Alberta, Edmonton, Canada

Carla Patterson, MSc, PhD, GD Bus
Associate Professor and Director of Research
School of Public Health
Queensland University of Technology, Australia

Kobkul Phancharoenworakul, PhD, RN
Dean, Faculty of Nursing
Mahidol University, Bangkok, Thailand

Richard W. Redman, PhD, RN
Associate Dean, Academic Affairs; and Professor, School of Nursing
University of North Carolina at Chapel Hill, USA

Rosalina A.P. Rodrigues, PhD, RN
Professor, College of Nursing
University of São Pãulo at Ribeirão Preto, Brazil

Callista Roy, PhD, RN, FAAN
Professor, School of Nursing
Boston College, Chestnut Hill, MA, USA

Gwen D. Sherwood, PhD, RN, FAAN
Professor and Executive Associate Dean, School of Nursing
The University of Texas Health Science Center at Houston, TX, USA

Lillie M. Shortridge-Baggett, EdD, RN, FAAN, FNAP
Professor and Director of International Affairs, Lienhard School of Nursing
Pace University, Pleasantville, NY, USA
and Department of Nursing Science
University of Utrecht, The Netherlands

Oliver Slevin, PhD, RN
Lecturer in Nursing and Director of DNSc Programme, School of Nursing
University of Ulster at Jordantown, UK

Leana Uys, PhD, RN
Professor, School of Nursing
University of KwaZulu-Natal, South Africa

Ann Whall, PhD, RN, FAAN
Professor, School of Nursing
University of Michigan, Ann Arbor, MI, USA

Jenifer Wilson-Barnett, PhD, RN
Professor and Dean, Nightingale School of Nursing
King's College, London, UK

Bettina J. Woodford, PhD
Communications Officer, Daniel J. Evans School of Public Affairs
University of Washington, Seattle, WA, USA

Preface

Doctoral education prepares an individual for a career of leadership in research, education, management and policy making. Doctoral education in nursing is fairly recent when compared with the history of PhD programmes in other fields. Nurses in the USA began enrolling in and completing doctoral programmes in the early 1930s, while their counterparts in other parts of the world only began to enjoy the privilege beginning in the 1960s. Doctoral programmes that focus on nursing science are an even more recent phenomenon and the development of such programmes mostly occurred in the 1970s and 1980s. Currently, most of the doctoral degrees in nursing are granted in the USA, the UK and Australia, and students from around the globe are able to take advantage of the numerous programmes offered in these countries. However, with the emergence of doctoral programmes in other parts of the world, such as in Thailand, Egypt, Japan, New Zealand and elsewhere, innovative local options are becoming more available for those who seek doctoral preparation.

This book is a milestone in international nursing doctoral education and a wonderful example of best practice in global collaboration. It is the brainchild of a fairly new organization that evolved from an informal US-based forum on doctoral education. From its earliest days, the International Network for Doctoral Education in Nursing was a fully international organization bringing together leaders as well as students to address issues in nursing doctoral education. Through much dialogue about the issues, challenges and goals of doctoral education in nursing, it became abundantly clear that the nursing community needed a text to both shape such a dialogue as well as reflect it, pointing the way for the future. One of the unique features of this volume is that its global perspective is truly reflected in the collaborative co-authorships representing different countries in almost every chapter. The authors are representative of nursing doctoral education in the five continents and are renowned specialists in this field. Their partnership in writing this book is a metaphor for doctoral education for the future. With the technological and information explosion that has permeated educational programmes in all corners of the world, new collaborative models should emerge to facilitate cross-national study and the attainment of higher levels of knowledge and skills for the benefit of patients, their families and communities.

Nursing education faces many challenges that require the collective wisdom of educators to devise innovative approaches for addressing them. Among the many challenges, I believe, there are three that are most pressing: (i) In what ways does doctoral education enhance the development and advancement of nursing knowledge? (ii) Does a schism still exist between nursing practice and nursing research? (iii) What is the status of financing and support of doctoral education and students in different countries? I will briefly address each of these challenges.

The essence of doctoral education is the preparation of leaders who will become the future scholars who can shape the nature of the discipline's knowledge and its advancement. This is the first challenge. It is through apprenticeship and mentorship experiences during doctoral study that disciplinary questions are formulated and investigated. However, if students do not get the opportunity for dialogue and to debate questions and findings that evolve from a nursing perspective, the questions they choose to investigate and the answers they uncover may not advance knowledge that bears on the nursing encounter or the health of clients. With the proliferation of doctoral programmes in many parts of the world, educators should ponder the question of whether or not nursing knowledge (theory, philosophy, practice and science) is fully reflected in the curriculum, in the scholarly dialogue encouraged in the programme, in the literature selected to inform the students, and the guidance they receive from faculty mentors. Do the questions asked and the evidence produced through the research process inform primarily the discipline of nursing and the quality of care outcomes or do they primarily inform other disciplines?

The second challenge is how to deal with the schism that has existed between nursing practice and nursing research for a long time. Nursing is among a number of fields that provide many options for those who graduate with a doctoral degree. It is precisely because of how educators have viewed practice, research, theory and their interrelationships that a variety of programmes were developed leading to a variety of degrees, such as the Doctor of Philosophy (PhD), Doctorate in Nursing Science (DNSc), Doctorate in Education in Nursing (EdD), the Nursing Doctorate (ND) and more recently (in the USA), a Practice Doctorate. This trend in multiple letters depicting the different degrees has led to confusion among the potential applicants to the various programmes, as well as among the employers of the graduates. The intent of these programmes is to offer options to enable graduates to focus on one role (educator, clinician, researcher) and to develop knowledge that is most congruent with that role. Whether this US model, emulated in different countries in various formats, is the best for our discipline should be debated. This approach, developed in the USA as a result of a highly decentralized educational system, has unwittingly perpetuated the research/practice/theory schism, and may not facilitate the interconnections between them. The fundamental relationships between practice, reseach and theory and the potential for creating a unified set of degrees should drive a stimulating international dialogue. Nursing will benefit from the wisdom now available in different countries where varying paradigms, opinions, as well as different educational environments have been developed for nursing doctoral education.

The third international challenge is the financing of doctoral education, doctoral research and doctoral students. Early in the history of graduate education in nursing, many countries provided different types and levels of support to programmes and students. Some countries continue to provide students with support in the form of scholarships, traineeships and sponsorships, either partial or full. However, the limited resources now being devoted to advanced degrees in nursing are reflecting shifts in the overall global economy, and the opportunities for such resources are diminishing. Simultaneously, doctoral programmes in nursing have achieved a degree of maturity, enabling them to become more rigorous and demanding, requiring full-time attention from students. How to financially support the students is a challenge that needs to be addressed by a global group of educators who have a passion for developing the best future nurse scientists. Shared sponsorships, and other ways of supporting students' research could be creatively designed to inspire and support future doctoral students. A similar concern relates to the availability of resources for programme and faculty support, which vary greatly across the many countries offering doctoral education.

Thinking globally about doctoral programmes in nursing is a step in the right direction. Learning from each other and developing strategies that evolve from the experience of educators from different parts of the world can provide a critical framework to address the increasing number of challenges and hurdles experienced by educators and doctoral students around the globe.

This book is an innovative and knowledgeable resource on doctoral education and will stimulate developing better solutions to problems and challenges that have existed for a long time. It is a must read for any student, faculty member, or administrator who is interested in higher education, and doctoral education specifically, in all parts of the world. While it does not reflect all types of doctoral programmes, it should stimulate the development of similar collections of writing around the globe. Its publication will change the landscape of the literature on nursing doctoral education.

Afaf I. Meleis
Professor and Dean
The University of Pennsylvania
School of Nursing
USA

Introduction

This book aims to reflect the state of doctoral education as it exists today internationally. It also aims to project future developments, based on knowledge of the present. For the past quarter century doctoral education has been transformed in most regions of the world, although the dynamics and particulars of *how* and *what* vary greatly as a function of the healthcare needs of populations, the state of nursing science and nursing education within countries, as well as political and other relevant social developments.

Thus it has been a challenge to try to capture the state of doctoral education worldwide; yet, the team of authors assembled for this book has been more than equal to this challenge. These authors are leaders in their own countries, having had substantial participation in, and influence on, doctoral education in their countries, bringing both breadth and depth to bear on the topic at hand. We are most grateful to them for their contributions and for the team spirit they brought to the enterprise of this book. Several other individuals served as key informants from their countries, providing information that was used in various chapters, expanding the scope of the chapters to incorporate information well beyond the settings of the particular authors. We are grateful to them as well.

Currently, doctoral education is offered in 31 countries. A listing of these appears in tabular form in Chapter 12 (see Table 12.1). Over the years visionary leaders have been instrumental in the expansion of doctoral education worldwide, as have international foundations and government agencies that have provided facilitation, resources and funding enabling the growth we see today. The talents of leaders will continue to be in great demand, as they face the challenge of addressing quality issues of doctoral education in their countries in the years ahead.

Since the formation of the International Network for Doctoral Education in Nursing (http://www.umich.edu/~inden/) and its formalization in 2000, we have endeavoured to learn about and describe the nature of doctoral education in various regions of the world. This turned out to be a process that continues today. We understand more about the nature of doctoral study in some regions than in others. Historically, nursing research and doctoral education have been inextricably linked together, and this is how it should be. In countries where nursing research has expanded in quantity and impact, so has doctoral education. Where research has been constrained, so has doctoral education. Conversely, where doctoral education has taken root, nursing research has flourished. Another development that has contributed to the exponential growth in doctoral education around the world has been collaboration among and between nursing scientists and leaders across national boundaries. Opportunities created for dialogue, exchange, collaboration, mutual influence, consultation and mentoring are reflected in positive ways in the developments in doctoral education we see today.

Our understanding of nursing science has evolved over the years. There was an assumption held previously that nursing science generated on a given topic in a particular setting or country should to be applicable to other countries and settings. We now know better. We now have a better grasp of the contextual nature of nursing science and its specificity. We have come to understand how the culture, history, the nature of illnesses and their trajectories, as well as populations with their richness and variability, make it well nigh impossible to transplant and use nursing science and nursing knowledge generated in one country to the situation in another. Thus, nursing scholars as well as funding agencies have emphasized collaborative research, and have come to value multi-site studies that promise to enhance the generalizability of research findings to other settings. Clearly, more needs to be done to understand better the healthcare problems that are seen in many parts of the world. However, nurse scientists in many countries of the world are constrained in their efforts to do research due to lack of resources and qualified personnel. The 10/90 disequilibrium was identified several years ago by the World Health Organization and others as a major problem in health research and it continues to be a compelling reality in many countries. This formulation is a dramatic way of expressing the problem that only 10% of research resources worldwide are spent on the health problems of 90% of the global population. Strategies to rectify this imbalance and inequity are being discussed on the world stage and will require that nurse scholars and leaders collaborate not only with one another across national boundaries, but with interdisciplinary colleagues as well and work at policy and political levels with governmental officials, as well as with international organizations and non-governmental groups. Nurse scholars in resource-rich countries can play a significant role in correcting this imbalance by studying and by guiding their doctoral students to study the health problems that are prevalent and debilitating for large populations in countries that lack the resources and collaborating with colleagues in these countries.

Doctoral education has experienced many changes over the years in response to national needs and the needs of those enrolled in doctoral study. For example, Australia has evolved a new doctoral degree and educational format for those nurses who prefer to stay in clinical settings and work with patients. Similarly, the UK has developed an alternative education path for younger nurses entering doctoral study whose background has been heavily clinical rather than as educators (the professional doctorate). On the surface the newer forms of doctoral study developed within Australia and the UK may seem similar but this is deceptive. Each new degree is uniquely suited to meet and respond to specific national needs and situations.

Within the USA innovation and debate have been ongoing since the inception of doctoral education in the 1930s. Variations have existed in degree designation, programme content, the expected 'product,' as well as the nature of the graduates and the competence expected of them upon completion of the programme. At the time of writing several institutions are introducing newer programme elements or new programme foci or even new degrees, with a view to preparing different types of graduate than those which have historically existed. One institution has embarked on a doctorate of nursing practice degree to prepare individuals for clinical leadership or executive leadership; another institution is proposing a doctorate of nursing practice to prepare nurses for expert level patient care in inpatient and outpatient settings to fill the gap created by the decline in primary care physicians; several nursing organizations are working together to propose a similar form of clinical doctorate to enable attainment of clinical competence beyond the Master's level through evidence-based inquiry, while the American Association of Colleges of Nursing has created a task force to study the professional clinical doctorate. Such apparent ferment and foment has something 'untidy' about it, but viewed from a historical perspective, can be seen as keeping the nursing doctoral education perpetually dynamic and evolving, rather than settled or static.

In response to different forces, changes have occurred in the approach to and format of doctoral education as well in its content. In an effort to reach multiple constituencies some schools have evolved their doctoral programme offerings to be taught online, through the internet, either partially or totally, making creative uses of technology to keep students and faculty in ongoing virtual contact. In other cases, where countries once sent their students overseas for doctoral study, educators have developed their own doctoral programmes, and are using the 'sandwich' concept, whereby students are supported to go overseas for a year during the middle period of their doctoral study. This enables students to benefit from research-intensive environments overseas, while staying grounded within their own country, developing research projects that are responsive to the healthcare needs of their own populations and staying much more sensitive to the at times questionable applicability of Western nursing theories and nursing science to their own cultural and national contexts. This strategy has the added benefit to the country of being much more economical in terms of expenditure of funds.

Viewed from a worldwide perspective, nursing doctoral education is thus like a rich and complex kaleidoscope, with many differences and variations, always evolving and undergoing change through evolution rather than revolution. It is this kaleidoscope that we aim to capture in this book.

The contents of the book are presented in two parts. In Part I, we focus on substantive issues: we begin with some philosophical discussion underpinning nursing science; we discuss the interconnections between nursing science/ research and doctoral education; we discuss how transformational leadership can be cultivated through doctoral education; we describe the Re-envisioning Project that has had so much impact, first beginning in the USA, and subsequently expanding to many countries; we address the dynamics of the marketplace and how these influence doctoral education; and finally, we discuss faculty shortage and how it can impact doctoral education.

In Part II we deal with the processes and operational issues in doctoral education, and the various elements involved in undertaking doctoral study. The chapters in this section deal with the doctoral process; the role of mentors; monitoring of quality; non-traditional and emergent forms of doctoral education; international exchange opportunities for doctoral students; postdoctoral study; and lastly, a chapter that presents a compilation of resources and funding opportunities for research and doctoral study, an area of critical importance to doctoral students.

In writing this book, it is our hope that it will contribute to the dialogue and debate on many of the issues addressed in the chapters. We also hope that it will stimulate others to contribute their voices to discussions of the future and how we might get there. We welcome input and comments from our readers.

Shaké Ketefian
Hugh P. McKenna

Chapter 1

The substance of doctoral education

Oliver Slevin and Somchit Hanucharurnkul

This first chapter is primarily concerned with the content of doctoral education in nursing now and in the future. In addressing this, it is necessary to consider the context within which such education takes place and the wider emerging trends that may influence future directions. We have identified three issues: the *content* of doctoral programmes; the *context* within which they develop; and *nursing* as the field of study in such programmes. The links and interrelationships between these will influence the structure and processes as well as the content of future doctoral preparation.

The problem with taking account of context is not only that it is by definition complex, but also that it is a constantly changing milieu. When faced with burgeoning change we are immediately drawn with urgency towards consideration of the future challenges and how we will respond to these. This can emerge as a sense of drivenness in respect of arriving at solutions. However, in such circumstances there is a risk that the fundamental nature of the phenomena under consideration and how they came to be may be overlooked. It is vitally important that the ground from which we move forward is not only fully understood but that the movement into the future takes full account of our past and the issues confronting us in the present. There are essentially two scenarios that may unfold, although it may be more appropriate to see these as extreme ends of a continuum. One road (and perhaps that most travelled) is to continue in a piecemeal fashion. The other represents an opportunity now given to us to reflect upon a more meaningful way forward.

In this chapter we will demonstrate that even on an international level there is a degree of commonality between doctoral programmes. However, there is also a great degree of variance and this is the case not only between nations but also between higher education institutions within nations. In the past, this has been a matter of some concern. However, as the pace of change increases, and as we attempt to change our doctoral programmes to maintain their relevance in a changing world, there is a greater risk of doctorates losing even that limited amount of international currency they presently enjoy. Here we cannot hope to present anything approximating to a master plan for the development of doctoral programmes in the new millennium, but perhaps we can outline the issues and in so doing contribute to that reflective dialogue.

In attempting to ensure that order emerges from the edge of chaos, there is perhaps at least one 'constant' to which we can hold. The foundational premise among all of the above considerations is that of nursing. Whatever we determine to be the purpose of doctorates and the nature and content of doctoral education, they are first and foremost *about* nursing. That is, we are concerned with the highest source of learning that will inform our practice. We have alluded already to the issue of historicity, how the past informs the present and how we must endeavour to bring the best of what we have learned into the future. We have long recognized the importance of establishing a sound body of theory that informs (and is informed by) our practice, in terms of what Dickoff and James (1968) termed 'situation producing theory' and Argyris and Schön (1974) later referred to as theory-of-action that would be enacted in 'theory-in-use'. Similarly, while we are well acquainted with the dangers of mindlessly following tradition in our practice, we nevertheless value the wisdom that has emerged through experience, as reflected by Benner and her colleagues (Benner, 1984; Benner et al, 1999). Such groundings must be adapted to future circumstances and supplemented by new knowledge. The nursing paradigm or worldview, in the sense originally posited by Kuhn (1970), is a dynamic and changing perspective, and much more so in a rapidly changing world. The current and future cohorts of doctoral nurses will be those most charged with meeting this challenge in the future. They are the creators, innovators, keepers and purveyors of the paradigm. It is therefore of vital importance that those so charged are adequately prepared for the task. This is the matter we must address here and throughout this book.

Fundamental issues

Nursing

Nursing and its mission must be the foundation of our future development of doctoral education. However, it is a characteristic of the foundationalist epistemology that a body of knowledge depends for its endurance upon the strength of its foundational premises. On this basis, the survival of our project depends on a strong and enduring conceptualization of the nature of nursing itself. Should this be unsound, the total edifice of nursing knowledge and practice that we construct through nursing scholarship (including doctoral and postdoctoral study) is unstable and in danger of collapse. We must, after all, know *what* doctoral education is intended to improve or advance. It is beyond the remit of this chapter to enter upon a lengthy discourse on the nature of nursing. This is a matter that has been addressed elsewhere. Within modern times, it is many years since Henderson's (1966) celebrated definition of nursing laid the groundwork of nursing as a service of helping those in need when they were unable to meet such needs themselves. Since then, many have made their contributions. Watson's (1990) seminal notion of 'informed moral passion', identifying the vital importance of the integrity and inter-relationships between best available knowledge and skills, ethical deportment and a commitment to concern and care for the other, admirably conveys the essential nature of nursing work. On a different level Slevin (1999) has spoken of 'nursing as a relationship that involves caring for others in a health context', bringing together the four metaparadigmatic elements of person (others), health, environment (context) and nursing (caring), previously identified by Fawcett (1984, 2000).

It might well be argued that this is going over old ground, that indeed there is no longer controversy or issues to resolve in this area. This might be true if nursing is considered to be synonymous with (or accurately reflected by) the voluminous academic nursing literature on the nature of nursing. However, if it is recognized that nursing is also in the nature of a social contract, whereby 'society' expects nursing to provide care of a particular form and nursing is in turn recognized and accepted to the extent that it meets this commission, all may not be well. For example, even in the closing weeks of 2003, in the United Kingdom (UK) there emerged two damning reports (Magnet, 2003; Sergeant, 2003). Both claim that nurses are failing their patients within the UK National Health Service (NHS), and that they all too often exhibit uncaring attitudes and fail to provide even the most fundamental aspects of physical and psychological care. Our doctoral education, and its content, will be of little value if it does not contribute to us seeing how nursing is and what it could become. Criticisms such as these typically argue that the preparation of nurses has become too academic, that the movement of nursing into higher education is the root cause of the failure to provide adequate preparation for practice. Nurses, so the argument runs, become more concerned with status, more involved in administrative tasks and specialized technical work, and less prepared to undertake what might be considered menial 'bed and body' work. Such arguments might extend to question the relevance of higher degrees in nursing, and the relevance of doctorates in particular.

Nature of a doctorate

It is helpful at this stage to briefly consider the idea of a doctorate. The term 'doctor' derives originally from the Latin *docere* meaning to show or to teach. Such teachings would be based primarily on the *doctrina*, the body of teachings. The 'doctor' or 'scholar' (derived from the Latin *scholasticus* or learned, and the Ancient Greek *skholastikos* or studious) was recognized as the producer *and* conveyor of such knowledge. Thus, the qualification of 'Doctor' (initially in theology and later in other professions) emerged from the Middle Ages as the highest degree of a university – the doctorate (with its most universal title being Doctor of Philosophy or PhD). Significantly, in later centuries, and particularly during the era of scientific positivism, there emerged the idea of science as a pure calling, concerned with the quest for truth and knowledge and not its practical and ethical implications. Postdoctoral scientists, active in research, tended to distance themselves from the social consequences of their work and even within the universities viewed teaching as a lesser activity to be tolerated if not indeed avoided. It is only in recent decades that the link between scholarship and teaching again emerged as an important concern.

There can of course be no rational argument against the education of nurses for a complex and often life-saving undertaking at an appropriate and advanced level. There may, however, be a recognition that such education *could* go astray, that there is indeed a possibility of failing to see the wood for the trees. It therefore becomes imperative that nursing as a profession develops a relevant body of knowledge and skills, that these are enhanced to meet changing needs, and that there is leadership for a way forward that is firmly grounded in knowledge and wisdom. It is the need for this grounding, and this wisdom, that is in fact the *raison d'être* for doctorates in nursing. The content of doctoral programmes, in terms not only of what this learning is but also how it is to be achieved, is therefore of vital importance.

Context

We have considered nursing as being a social contract between 'society' and the profession. This is a sense in which we must respond to the needs of those we would care for. These needs are complex and demanding when they are expressed in the wants of public opinion. The demands placed upon nursing are at once imposed by governments and their political agendas for health, yet in a sense transcend party politics and time. There are calls (as in the papers by Magnet (2003) and Sergeant (2003)) for nursing to be not only a stabilizing and humanizing constant in an increasingly complex and alienating healthcare world, but also a challenge to modernize in the face of rapid change and technological advancement.

The nurse at the bedside faces the demands of the moment, within that culture and that setting, constrained by the policy of the wider institution and even by the wider conditions of national policy. However, increasingly, influences from the even wider global milieu press in upon this situation. Where this 'bedside' is in a developing country, the scarcity imposed by multinational pharmaceutical strategies, international trade restrictions and global harm factors are very real threats to the wellbeing and even survival of the person being nursed. In the developed countries, the 'patient' and/or the 'nurse' at this bedside – whether it be in New York, London or Paris – are now likely to have emerged from another culture, so that the actual delivery of care is now almost always transcultural in its delivery.

All these influences point up the third linking factor we propose, that of *context*. Insofar as nursing will be influenced by context (and possibly act as an influencing force within its context), the nature and content of doctoral education will similarly be influenced (and possibly equally influential). In a multicultural and global world the construction of knowledge and practice can no longer be unidimensional and bounded exclusively to a particular culture and its values. In the remainder of this chapter, we consider the impact of context and the implications of this for the content of doctoral programmes in nursing.

Trends that will affect doctoral education

Questions begged

What is good about doctoral education? What is bad about doctoral education? How will doctoral preparation evolve in the future? These questions are amenable to comparatively straightforward answers. Yet these are questions that have been posed before, certainly over some decades in the previous century, with little emerging in the way of clarity. Despite such ongoing dialogue, there has been no significant shift in the nature of doctoral education over these decades. Aware as we are that the world has changed significantly, especially in the two decades spanning the new millennium, it is reasonable to assume that the challenges faced by those who have undertaken doctoral preparation will also have changed dramatically. If this *is* the case, then serious questions must indeed be asked about the apparent lack of development in how such individuals are prepared. This is no less the case in respect of nursing, where what nurses do has a direct impact on the health and wellbeing, and indeed survival, of those they serve.

The questions now begged must therefore be: What is so different about this time? Why should our inquiries lead to anything more than maintenance of the *status quo* now? Part of the answer to these questions resides in the awareness that the world is rapidly changing, and our responses must change as well. It is many years since Alvin Toffler (1970) introduced the idea that the world is changing at such a rapid rate that we experience a sense of lack of control, a feeling of alienation, an awareness of our vulnerability – a phenomenon he described as *future shock*. More than a decade after Toffler had written, Naisbitt (1984) in his almost equally famous statement mapped out with extraordinary clarity the trends starting to emerge – including the movement from an industrial to an information age and the shift from national to world economies.

However, what may be different now is how change not only advances with increasing rapidity, but the way in which the consequences of such change are now starting to turn in upon us. We are confronted with the limitations of science in terms of its erstwhile apparent promise of a new utopia. Even those at the forefront of our sciences recognize the illusion of order in the face of chaos, and the limitations of science beyond certain points (Horgan, 1996; Barrow,

1998). But of even greater concern is the fact that while the advances in scientific knowledge have brought great advantages, we are now becoming conscious of the great damage and high risks of the often unanticipated negative impacts of these advances on local and global levels (Beck, 1999; Giddens, 1999).

Complexity

What, then, are the trends that are of particular concern to doctoral preparation in general and *nursing* doctoral preparation in particular? To a large extent these are made more complex by the fact that the trends are interrelated. In a sense, this is perhaps the fundamental and underlying change, often referred to in the scientific literature as *complexity theory* (Waldrop, 1992). The real world is complex, fuzzy and unpredictable. In the sense originally posited by David Bohm (1980), meaning is *enfolded* in the wholeness of what he termed the implicate order. In our attempts at *unfoldment*, at deriving meaning, we are at once faced with the danger of fragmentation – the illusion that the fragments we see through particular worldviews or lenses are in fact the *real* world. The project is further compromised by the fact that what is enfolded is dynamic and forever changing. This therefore becomes an issue of not so much *what* we think, but *how* we think. Old formulae no longer work, and there is a need to be more reflexive in seeking new ways to solve new problems that often have no precedents. It is increasingly the case that no single lens (or discipline) can satisfactorily address problems that are so enfolded and multidimensional.

This fact has implications for new physics and economics, as illustrated by Waldrop (1992), and it is no less important in nursing. Here also we are faced with fuzzy worlds and complex, rapidly changing situations: acquired immune deficiency syndrome/human immunodeficiency virus, elder care, suicide, are but a few examples. However we deliver our nursing doctorates in the future, one thing is certain: we will not be able to depend exclusively on old formulae for solving new problems. While the traditional starting principles and skills of inquiry may form the bases of such programmes, the capacity to respond to new situations with new modes of inquiry will be a vital ingredient. And many of the issues we must resolve will not be amenable to single worldviews, unidisciplinary perspectives, or even uni-national modes of inquiry.

Beyond the premise of complexity, there are indeed other trends that may be of importance. These might in general fall under the following headings:

- Modernity
- Consequent changes in healthcare systems
- Globalization
- The professional response

Modernity

The modern condition

In North America the influential work of Charles Taylor (1991) drew attention to the crisis of what he termed the ethics of authenticity – the negative impact of the modern condition upon the way we live. He spoke of the three malaises: increasing individualism where, while there is individual choice and freedom, there is also the demise of a stable order and a communitarian consciousness; the impact of instrumental reasoning and ways in which science and technology are in one sense liberating and empowering, but in another sense disempowering and increasingly create designed environments that place limits on our freedom of choice; and the increasing lack of confidence and engagement in the modern politic as, individualized and isolated, people become 'enclosed in their own hearts'. As was the case for the old religions with their claim to establishing a sacred order in society, so too has the new age of science and technology failed to create a modern utopia. We do of course have the advantages of modern science and technology, and nowhere is this more evident than in the field of healthcare. But as we have entered a new millennium, the risks incurred by failure to control advances in science and technology threaten our very existence on the planet (Beck, 1992, 1997).

The postmodern turn

One consequence of what became known as the postmodern turn, particularly as it progressed towards the final decades of the past century, was its increasingly critical stance in relation to the given order of things. The works of Jean-Francois Lyotard (1984) and Michel Foucault (1970) were significant drivers in this postmodern approach. In essence, the perspective is represented by a sceptical critique of any perspective whose discourse seeks to explain the world, what Lyotard described as 'incredulity towards metanarratives'. The postmodern legacy of scepticism – in essence a questioning and critical attitude – was a significant influence upon late twentieth century thinking in all walks of life, including nursing (Watson, 1999). However, this critical stance contained its own inbuilt demise. Postmodernism also required a sceptical attitude to any claims it might itself make in respect of a response to the limits and excesses of modernity. The movement offered only a critical response, but no solution to the failures it identified; such claims would in turn be subject to the circularity of postmodern criticism, in that any constructive way forward emerging from a postmodern discourse would itself be subject to critical deconstruction. It was therefore for others to propose new ways forward. These new ways have been contained within movements variously termed late modernity or new modernity (Beck, 1999, 2000; Giddens, 1999, 2001; Giddens and Hutton, 2000). The basic tenets of such positions run as follows: in a new world characterized by burgeoning change, increased risks, and an increasingly global consciousness, the solutions and formulae of the past no longer hold. As new technologies of modernity emerge and advance at an increasing rate, the discourse has moved from one of hailing in an unconditional way how we are moving towards a new utopia, to a recognition that the technologies of the past and those now emerging present major threats to our very existence. We realize, perhaps too late, that the major challenges of the future will include how we contain the risks we have ourselves manufactured. We are, in effect, entering a new world that demands of us new-think responses. This is of profound importance in respect of how we will prepare the most able among us to confront the challenges of the future. Here too there comes a realization that while doctoral education for nurses in the future may find some historical firm ground from which to push forward, the greater demand will be that of preparing our thinkers of the future for responding to new and changing situations with new and different modes of inquiry.

Changes in healthcare systems

The advances of modernity impact with particular effect on our healthcare systems. Advances in science and technology are nowhere more dramatic than in the field of healthcare. There are the impacts of the harmful or threatening effects of modernity – ranging from the malaises identified by Taylor (1991) to the more concrete impact of pollution (from chemicals, emissions and radiation), through the demands on resources imposed by increased longevity, to 'new' healthcare problems ranging from AIDS to obesity. It is true that the discoveries of new and more effective antibiotics and antiseptics throughout the twentieth century saved hundreds of millions of lives. However, as we move into the twenty-first century these same substances create new 'superbugs' that may even threaten humanity.

Also impacting upon our healthcare systems are the rapid increases in information and technology. There is the possibility of *knowing* more and better, and of technology allowing us to *do* more than we perhaps ever dreamed. But even here, there is a sense in which modernity turns back upon us. In the quest for quality, we aspire to health services that provide safe and effective services based upon the modern-day mantra of evidence-based medicine (EBM) and its fellow travellers (evidence-based practice, evidence-based nursing, evidence-based healthcare). But such is the speed and volume of information production and technology advancement that the capacity to ascertain the quality of the product, disseminate it and effectively incorporate it into clinical practice, is almost insurmountable (Baker, 1998).

The sum of these trends can be viewed in terms of a net increase in demand – for more and better services – set against a constant increase in scarcity of resources. In the developing nations the scarcity of resources is absolute and more often than not life threatening. However, even in the developed nations this has become a crucial issue. Despite the fact that over 90% of healthcare provision is concentrated in the richest nations, the demand continues to outstrip the resources.

It is within this real-world scenario that nursing must find its place and meet its commitment to best purpose. We need to know how *we* will cope with changing patterns of health and healthcare delivery. We need to establish what evidence is needed for *our* best practice, and how this is best disseminated and implemented. Furthermore, we must also establish how *nursing* will respond to the ethical dilemmas that are already appearing in the developed *and* developing world, as demand outstrips supply. Importantly, we must also recognize that these complex and multidimensional concerns cannot be addressed exclusively from a nursing perspective. We speak much today of multidisciplinary care and teamwork. In promoting such an orientation, we recognize the importance of shared education and training. But behind and underpinning these orientations is a need to recognize the importance of multidisciplinary approaches to research and the need to incorporate such an orientation and the particular attitudes and competencies required within doctoral preparation.

Globalization

Of particular importance in the thrust of modernity is the phenomenon that has become known as globalization. The term is the subject of much use and indeed abuse, meaning different things to different people. In general, it contains somewhere within it a closing down of space and differences as a consequence of developments in new technologies, particularly those involving high technology communication and rapid-transit travel. Not only is the entire globe aware of and contributing to the exchange of global information, but it is also possible to physically traverse the globe in less than a day. By the end of the 1990s there was a lauding of economic globalization (with the institution of the World Trade Organization (WTO) and the credo of free trade), and the major powers were adopting a global consciousness within which they viewed themselves as the caretakers of the new global stage. However, contained within this trend are the threats emerging from our failure to recognize the risks involved. This was powerfully expressed by Capra, when he stated:

> As this new century unfolds, it becomes increasingly apparent that the neoliberal 'Washington Consensus' and the policies and economic rules set forth by the Group of Seven and their financial institutions – the World Bank, the IMF and the WTO – are consistently misguided. Analyses by scholars and community leaders . . . show that the 'new economy' is producing a multitude of interconnected harmful consequences – rising social inequality and social exclusion, a breakdown of democracy, more rapid and extensive deterioration of the natural environment, and increasing poverty and alienation. The new global capitalism has also created a global

> criminal economy that profoundly affects national and international economies and politics; it has threatened and destroyed local communities around the world; and with the pursuit of an ill-conceived biotechnology it has invaded the sanctity of life by attempting to turn diversity into monoculture, ecology into engineering and life itself into a commodity.
>
> (Capra, 2002, p. 181)

It is perhaps unsurprising that Beck (2002) also links such developments to the emergence of global terror, and in turn the way in which this not only brings threats to communities from without, but also a new consciousness of fear and confinement within.

It may be the case that to some extent those such as Giddens, Beck and Capra are excessive and unreasonable in their claims. And there is certainly a case for introducing balance, by recognizing the great successes science, technology and international relations have sometimes brought in the previous century. Notwithstanding this, we must also recognize that the global threats we now face do to some extent emerge from a range of failures, including:

- the incapacity to anticipate or take adequate action to avert the negative effects of modern developments such as fossil fuel and nuclear energy usage
- the failure to control the impact of scientific and technological advances in increasingly complex situations that result in increasing risks to health and wellbeing, within and across national boundaries
- the introduction of economic models that, while having the appearance of sophistication, were in reality based upon values of profit and vested interest that served to widen inequalities, increase global poverty and create new health risks
- the failure to accompany global development with a global ethic that reflects values of global justice and communal concerns
- the resulting backlash of a destabilized global politic, which includes a new threat of global terrorism.

We have already noted how modernity and its risks, in and of themselves, require such new orientations. But now we find that the changes taking place, the information explosion and its rapid transmission, the impact of technology, the emerging risks, and the responses demanded are increasingly global. They confront not only national governments, industry and commerce, societies and the global community of the future but also the academic community of scholars and researchers. Significantly, knowledge is no longer localized and bound to particular contexts. It is shared and transmitted globally, not only influencing others in other settings but also being adapted by them and reflected back upon its origins. In their seminal work on how thought (as a source) emerges, Deleuze and Guattari (1987) spoke of nomadic thought (now often spoken of as nomadic theory). According to this, a theory has an origin, a distance traversed, a set of conditions for acceptance or rejection, and finally a transformed (incorporated) idea occupying a new position in a new time and place. The difference now, in the global era, is the extent to which an element of reflexivity and non-linearity enters upon this process. Now, the transformed thinking (or theory) is turned back on its origins, where it is in turn transformed. Edward Said (2000) spoke of this as travelling theory, influencing and being influenced. Thus, something as fundamental as gender and equality may transfer from the USA to a Muslim Far Eastern country and be interpreted in that location. Such interpretation is now reflected back upon northern England, impacting not only upon the Anglo-Saxon population but also the large Muslim community in that location.

We see in such processes the extent to which academic study has now also truly reached global dimensions. The non-linear ways in which knowledge is constructed are no less relevant to nursing than to other areas of academic endeavour. Indeed, it might be argued that in a world facing the global threats referred to by Capra (2002) nursing can be a vital force in infusing a caring and compassionate dimension in a world increasingly threatened by the politics of power and the ethics of utility. This is witnessed, for example, in the International Council of Nurses (1999) courageous stand in decrying the trend of developed countries attempting to remedy their own nursing shortages by recruiting from areas of great need in the developing countries. Significantly, the Global Advisory Group on Nursing and Midwifery (established by the World Health Assembly in the early 1990s) has emerged as a recognition of the vital role nurses can play on the world stage (World Health Assembly, 1996, 2001). When we now speak of a community of scholars, and more specifically a community of *nursing* scholars, we increasingly must see this as a global community where collaborative working and sharing crossing national boundaries and cultures may become the norm. It might be argued that what we have here is an imperative for revolutionary changes in nursing doctoral education that encompass this global dimension.

The professional response

Thus far we have recognized the importance of a firm disciplinary foundation from which nursing must move forward. And we have recognized also that one aspect of this is accepting that nursing is by definition contextual and relational. That is, nursing in the past, in the present, and in the future has and will continue to be a social construction influenced by trends within the wider world in which nursing takes place. We have considered some of these trends in the previous sections: increasing complexity; modernity and its risks; the emergence of health and healthcare patterns in the modern age; and the increasing global nature of these trends. However, it is important to avoid a deterministic outlook that sees nursing as being exclusively *reactive* in its response to such trends. There is a sense in which nursing must also be *proactive* in determining how the profession will not only respond to such influences but also how it will shape itself to serve more effectively in the future.

It is important to recognize that the changes now taking place beg questions in respect of the shape our profession will take in the future. Insofar as nursing sees itself as a profession, it is important to reflect briefly upon how this is perceived. A consideration of the etymological roots of the terms is of help. There are two root terms of importance here, both of Latin origin. The Latin word *professio* refers to a public declaration and it is the root word of the term 'profess' or 'I profess'. The Latin word *vocatio* refers to a calling or calling out. Originally, it related to a calling from God to perform some duty or take up some position. Thus we have the first great or high profession: that of divinity or the church. To a call from God, some professed publicly their response to enter into this service.

Carr-Saunders (1955), in what is widely considered the most famous position on the nature of a profession, added two other great professions that also emerged in antiquity: law and medicine. In respect of these three (church, medicine and law), they consisted of learned men, recognized as being possessed of knowledge and skill in a special area of work, and charged with and devoted to the service of others. Slevin (2003a) has suggested that these elements or properties of a profession can be identified in terms of certain rights and obligations: *delegated rights*, that *include autonomy*, *monopoly*, *and rewards*; and *accepted obligations*, that include expertise, integrity, and service.

The extent to which nursing has achieved these professional attributes is one of ongoing debate. It is certainly recognized that nursing has aspired to such status. In this respect, it might be recognized that it has met its professional *obligations*: nursing might claim to have achieved a degree of expertise attained through higher education; it has certainly (at least in most developed countries) met a condition of integrity by vesting its moral obligations in sophisticated professional codes of conduct; and it might claim to meet the condition of 'service' insofar as care is delivered effectively and in accordance with defined standards. However, on the issue of *rights* the situation is less clear. It is generally recognized that nurses do not have autonomy except in a few circumscribed situations. It would be hard to identify aspects of the diffuse range of nursing activities that could truly be seen as monopolistic, or exclusive to the work of qualified nurses.

Amongst all these professional attributes, that of autonomy is particularly important in determining professional status in the classical meaning of this term. It seems clear that no matter how far nursing may progress in other respects, the likelihood of achieving true autonomy within the context of how health services have been structured and delivered is remote. This situation is powerfully recognized, e.g. by Walsh (2000), and others such as Johnson (1972), Parry and Parry (1979) and Hugman (1998) have described a lesser position for which alternative terms such as 'mediated', 'agency' or 'bureau' profession have been concocted.

The aspiration of achieving professional status (in the traditional sense) would in any case require of nursing that it accepts a particular form of advanced knowledge and particular orientations towards maintaining autonomy, demanding monopoly, adopting moral positions and interpreting the notion of 'service'. In general, these are characteristically rational, logical, empirical, framed in problem-solving outlooks and typically assertive. It would indeed be remiss of nursing, as a predominantly female profession, if we did not also acknowledge the feminist insights behind this discussion, as addressed by Savage (1987), Davies (1995), Slevin (1999) and Walsh (2000). There is a sense in which the clinical detachment and case orientation of the medical profession is part of a wider masculine orientation, and as such, alien to the compassionate 'person-centredness' of the nursing project. There may of course be other professional groups who can avoid attaching a premium to the caring dimension of their work. But for nursing, this is not an option. Caring is a fundamental issue for nursing, it amounts to our *raison d'être*. A professional profile that engenders dispassion rather than compassion, clinical coldness rather than human warmth, detachment rather than connection, cannot be an option.

In entering the professional discourse, nursing must itself have a clear sense of the direction *it* wishes to take – not in terms of its own self-interest but in terms of the interests of those nursing represents, its patients or clients. It is astonishing that this very question was begged almost 20 years ago by Salvage, and we have not as yet succeeded in answering it. She stated:

> Nurses should not go along with the assumption that winning professional status for nurses would mean nothing but good for nurses and patients . . . Even if it could be proved that nursing did fulfil the criteria, nothing would change. We would still be as badly paid, and powerless, and patient care would not change. The question we should ask is not 'Is nursing a profession?' but 'Should we want nursing to be a profession, and if so, what do we mean by it? What are we hoping to achieve, and is this the best way of going about it?'
>
> (Salvage, 1985, p. 92)

The trends we have considered create urgency for now arriving at an answer to these questions. A more informed public has begun to question and indeed openly criticize the old monolithic notion of profession. The postmodern turn to which we referred earlier no doubt heralded this critical stance. As the limits of science have become more transparent, as access to information has become more readily available, and particularly as the negative effects of modernity become apparent, there is an unwillingness to mindlessly accept professional monopoly of knowledge and total autonomy in respect of decisions important to individuals and communities. The established professions are having to contemplate major shifts in their position within the modern world. Nursing can no longer turn to the old notions of what a profession is to inform how it will meet its responsibilities in the future. We are drawn back once again to Salvage's (1985) question. Those who will lead in the first decades of this new millennium must seek alternative professional orientations that more appropriately respond to the challenges of a new world. Old claims to autonomy and monopoly, and old forms of knowledge and knowledge construction will no longer hold. The demands of the new age point more towards involvement, empowerment and negotiation with those we serve, and the seeking of new ways to address new problems.

Implications for doctoral preparation in nursing

It will be clear from the previous section that there are a number of trends confronting nursing in the new millennium. This chapter is confined to addressing what might be considered the most important of these. They are issues that are relevant to the profession as a whole. However, the matter of *how* we address these issues is of vital importance. The decisions made must be based on a highly informed discourse. The responsibility for informing this discourse rests with those we might identify as nursing scholars. The preparation of such scholars is encompassed within doctoral programmes. The issue now confronting us is the form these programmes will take in the future.

In considering this issue it is useful to summarize the position as presented in the previous sections, in terms of the emerging trends and their implications for doctoral education. Based upon these considerations there are perhaps eight significant aspects that must be considered in establishing the nature, structure and content of future doctoral education.

1 *Establishing the theoretical and practice basis for advancement.* It is important that nursing establishes and affirms its body of theory and practice, and arrives at a shared paradigm as a sound springboard for moving forward.
2 *Taking account of context.* Nursing must be recognized as a relational activity that takes place within social contexts, ranging from intimate interpersonal relationships to global dimensions. Being in essence a social contract between those caring and those cared for, the future of nursing will emerge from these relations rather than any insular and inward-thinking processes.
3 *Recognizing complexity.* In developing its knowledge and theoretical base, nursing must recognize the limitations of linear thinking and the dangers of fragmented worldviews inherent in traditional ways of thinking. More reflexive approaches to seeking new ways of addressing new problems, rather than assuming old formulae will suffice, must be developed.
4 *Adopting a critical stance.* It is important that nursing becomes more conscious of dominant discourses that impose excessively rationalistic and instrumental ways of being that may not adequately address the knowledge and practice base essential to effective nursing. This will involve a more

sceptical orientation towards discourses that are essentially gendered and impose a unimodal scientific orientation that excludes alternative patterns of knowing and being.

5 *Harnessing the forces of modernity.* Adopting the aforementioned critical stance should not amount to an unreasoned and irrational rejection of the vast improvements that science and technology have brought to the modern world and in particular healthcare. It is important that society as a whole controls the way in which such developments advance the wellbeing of humankind, and that the risks emerging from such developments are minimized. Nursing must also embrace these opportunities and address the emerging risks.
6 *Sustaining and enhancing quality within modern healthcare settings.* It is important that nursing, in the aforementioned harnessing of modernity develops its own practices on the basis of best available evidence. This requires recognizing that within the wider context of evidence-based healthcare, there is a need for ensuring that the body of evidence for nursing is also advanced. But it also requires a recognition that problems of health and wellbeing do not fit neatly into unidisciplinary modes of thinking and that such issues must be addressed from a multidisciplinary perspective – in terms of how we think, learn *and* practice.
7 *Developing a global nursing consciousness.* As globalization advances, there is a need to recognize not only the impact of what happens in one nation upon all others, but also how the impact of the global influence of all nations now impacts upon each one. The specific health implications of these trends upon nursing must be confronted. However, of equal importance the potential of an emerging nursing global consciousness as a humanizing influence upon an increasingly alienating and threatening world must also be maximized.
8 *The creation of a new professional orientation.* In the past nursing has aspired to a professional status without a full appreciation of the implications of this aspiration or its relevance to nursing. It becomes increasingly clear that the old notions of a profession are inadequate for the new age. Instead, a more appropriate model must be developed, that emphasizes facilitative, empowering and negotiative aspects of a professional–client relationship, within which complex and often new problems are resolved in partnership.

The content of doctoral education

Unsteady foundations and uncertain futures

A doctoral programme is a preparation in research. All are agreed on this. However, in a changing world there are perhaps grounds for reflecting on what this means. There is a sense in which this means training to be a researcher. In the past, the student learned how to do a specific kind of research in a specific area of work, and usually within the confines of a graduate school or laboratory. On completion, the student would work in an academic institution or in a commercial laboratory setting, doing work the same as or similar to what he or she had been trained for. Sometimes, in the academic setting, the researcher would also teach, but little in the way of preparation for this was involved, at least during doctoral preparation. Issues of values or moral dilemma were not a concern, beyond those that would come under the rubric of research ethics (issues of informed consent, standards in respect of work with human or animal subjects, etc.). For the future, this will not do. As society-wide consciousness of the impact of the product of research, both positive and negative, upon our modern world increases, there are also arguments emerging about other concerns that should be addressed in such programmes. For example, those who undertake such programmes will need to take account of the impact of their work on the real world, and the impact of this world on how research should be conducted in the future. Indeed, as was suggested earlier, the new world of global modernization presents new threats and challenges that may even demand that different types of research work are carried out in very different ways. Doctoral preparation must change. The question is, how?

On the basis of our earlier discussion of emerging trends, it seems likely that now, much more than previously, there may be a willingness to countenance, and indeed adopt, new approaches to doctoral education. There is evidence that this is the case. However, the point reached in this process is unclear and there is currently considerable variability across the international stage. The degree of confusion is increased by the fact that not only do doctoral programmes vary from country to country, but also that this is in part a result of the overall variations in educational systems of which doctoral education is one end-point. Examples of such variations (the descriptions are not specific to nursing) include:

- In the USA, PhD programmes have typically extended over four years' full-time study and included an assessed coursework element. While apprenticeship or mentorship has been a significant element, this has not always been standardized. Assessment would typically be by defending a thesis to a panel.
- In the UK, PhD programmes have traditionally extended over three years' full-time study, excluded an assessed coursework element (although sometimes requiring entry following a master's degree), and functioned largely on master-and-apprentice models. Students are typically admitted as undifferentiated research students and assessed as meeting the standard (or otherwise) for doctoral study at the end of the first full-time year of study or its equivalent. In instances where the standard is not reached, the student proceeds to a master's level research degree (usually entitled MPhil) or withdraws. Assessment would typically be by presentation of a thesis and viva (oral) examination by an internal and external examiner.

- In France the PhD (known as the Doctorat), can only be embarked upon following a master's level programme where coursework is intensive and formally assessed, and requires four years of study. Assessment is by an internal panel of examiners followed by a public defence of the thesis.

Notwithstanding such differences, the international similarities in doctoral preparation outweigh national differences. Such programmes represent the most advanced level of tertiary or higher education, and in all situations their primary focus is the preparation of researchers or those for whom research or its application will be a significant aspect of their future careers. By the same token, in all situations the problems faced are similar. That is, the question of appropriateness of the PhD for meeting the challenges of the modern world.

Changing the gold standard

Concerns about the extent to which the PhD has adequately prepared researchers have led to increasing efforts to improve such programmes, and this has often included 'taught' elements. However, there is great variation from institution to institution in terms of the amount of student support. In some instances this is limited to what is provided within the supervisor–student relationship, while in others there is a more formal programme that often includes formally assessed elements. As indicated above, the inclusion of a coursework or taught element in the PhD programme is a standard approach in the USA, and in other countries the requirements for progression are also highly structured. While this has not been the case in the UK, here also there is a recognition of the need for greater attention to the organization of learning within the doctoral programme.

Significantly, within PhD programmes, where coursework *is* an element of the programme, the emphasis is on a more systematic underpinning to research issues – capacity for analytic and critical thinking, an understanding of the research process, the addressing of methodological issues, means of systematically reviewing literature, training in research design and methods, data analysis, report writing, etc. Augmenting these intellectual and research skills, in the past 15–20 years, PhD programmes in the USA have included content in various areas of nursing science that corresponds to national health priorities and/or faculty research expertise. While there is no national standard within the UK, guidelines issued by the Quality Assurance Agency (QAA) for Higher Education (the national body charged with monitoring and assuring higher education quality) provide a broad framework that institutions *may* utilize. The proposals for training in terms of coursework content are listed in Box 1.1. Notably, these proposals do extend the range of skills beyond those narrowly concerned with the conduct of research. However, the wording still conveys a narrowly instrumental approach that could not be construed as the extension of broader educational preparation into doctoral education.

Box 1.1 QAA skills training in research degrees

In considering the provision of skills training, institutions will wish to consider the development of:

- a broad understanding of the context in which the research takes place
- analytical and research skills, including the understanding of project design and research methodologies, appropriate to the subject and programme of study
- general and employment-related skills including, for example, interpersonal and team-working skills
- project management, information retrieval and database management, written and oral presentational skills, career planning and advice and intellectual property rights management
- language support and academic writing skills
- training and support for those researchers who may be involved in teaching and demonstrating activities

Quality Assurance Agency (1999)

In the USA, the American Association of Colleges of Nursing (AACN) similarly issues guidance in respect of PhD/DNSc (Doctor of Nursing Science) programmes (Box 1.2). However, in this instance, which relates specifically to nursing, the range of coursework is broader and encompasses professional as well as research-orientated areas of study. Significantly, while this guidance does recognize the importance of nursing and what is termed 'supporting content' does not exclude a wider educational dimension, this does indicate knowledge that may be construed as lacking in a broader global dimension. Nevertheless, a preparation based upon such guidance would address wider historical, philosophical and knowledge construction issues than found in other countries such as the UK. In addition, this guidance extends beyond the guidance within the UK's QAA guidance by recognizing the need to address practice and policy issues.

Box 1.2 AACN guidance on doctoral preparation

Core and related course content – the distribution between nursing and supporting content is consistent with the mission and goals of the program, and the student's area of focus and course work is included in:

- historical and philosophical foundations to the development of nursing knowledge
- existing and evolving substantive nursing knowledge
- methods and processes of theory/knowledge development
- research methods and scholarship appropriate to inquiry
- development related to roles in academic, research, practice or policy environments

American Association of Colleges of Nursing (2001)

While there are differences in the above two sets of guidelines, it is notable that in both instances there is a recognition that doctoral education must extend beyond its previous narrow orientation of subject-bound research training within a particular research paradigm. Clearly, while this is not explicitly stated, there is recognition that the demands of a changing world create corresponding demands for changes in how doctoral candidates are prepared. Indeed, this is part of a wider trend towards considering the international currency of higher education qualifications in general, including doctoral preparation. One notable instance of this is the movement within the European Community towards more standardized approaches. This is particularly reflected in the Bologna Declaration published by the European Ministers of Education in 1999. There is a commitment to establishing clarity and consistency across nations in terms of what is termed undergraduate and graduate cycles of educational preparation. However, as will also be noted, there is a commitment to what is termed a European dimension to be promoted in curricula and other educational activities (European Ministers of Education, 1999).

Innovative departures

As interest in doctoral education has advanced, various issues (perceived deficits in PhD, desired 'product', innovative approaches, etc.) have led to a rather confusing scenario. Much of this centres around the efficacy of the research programme, and this of course relates in large part to its goals in each case. One useful contribution is the 'empirical taxonomy' of doctorates proposed by the UK Council for Graduate Education (UKCGE), as presented in the following list (Bones, 2002):

- PhD by research
- PhD by publications
- New route PhD/advanced PhD/PhD plus
- Taught doctorate
- Professional doctorate
- Doctor of Medicine

The notion of a 'taught doctorate', i.e. one that largely consists of taught and assessed course elements, has tended to be unpopular in the UK, where the view that all doctorates are essentially research orientated holds sway. While a need for more educational input and training in research methods has been recognized, alternatives such as enhancing the PhD programme (new route PhD, PhD plus, etc.) that maintain the doing of research as the main activity are preferred. The Doctor of Medicine degree is usually specific to the medical profession and has similarities to the notion of a professional doctorate in other professions. As a consequence, the broad division emerging is between those described as PhD/DPhil (which in the UK can be achieved by research or publications) and the professional doctorate route. It is worth noting in passing that in the UK, within nursing, the professional doctorate is commonly described as a Doctor of Nursing Science (DNSc) degree. In the USA, degrees of this title are most often highly research focused and aligned with the PhD route, with a doctorate that has a more professional orientation being termed Nursing Doctorate (ND).

The idea of a professional doctorate is essentially that it will meet the needs of professionals whose main aspiration is the application of research within practice settings (McKenna and Cutcliffe, 2001). Such individuals aspire to leadership, managerial, advanced practice or educational roles rather than roles as career researchers within universities or research organizations (unlike in the USA, a doctorate in nursing education as a separate route has not emerged in the UK). While this has been the main form of innovative departure in doctoral education outside of developments within the PhD route itself, there is unfortunately a lack of consensus about the nature the variation should take. There is also a concern within the UK, Taiwan and Australia that professional doctorates may not have the same degree of international currency and credibility as the longer established PhD route. This is also an issue in the USA, as reported by Carpenter and Hudacek (1996). The different types of doctorate are described in detail elsewhere in this volume. The main features of such programmes are outlined below (drawn from various sources: Lunt, 2002; Higher Education Funding Council for England (HEFCE), 2003; Slevin, 2003b).

- They are Research Degree Programs (RDPs).
- They are formally recognized by governmental and accrediting bodies.
- There is normally a substantive formal taught component.

- They tend to be designed to meet the professional needs of students who are at levels of advanced standing within their professions.
- While such doctorates are *research* degrees, there is generally a broader conception of scholarship involved.
- There is an issue of whether professional doctorates in all cases produce new knowledge or extend current knowledge, or whether the application of research to practice is the more important criterion.
- Such programmes invariably involve the student/participant in activities of research or scholarly inquiry.
- There tends to be more flexibility and innovativeness in how these demands are expressed within programmes.
- The focus on flexibility and innovativeness is sometimes carried through to assessment, which may involve assessment of taught learning elements as well as theses, and may involve senior professionals in the learning support *and* assessment.

The context within which these programmes have developed is also one that increasingly is concerned with matters of quality. This has particularly been the case since the commencement of the millennium. In the UK, the Scottish Higher Education Funding Council (SHEFC) commenced this with the influential consultation entitled *Research and the knowledge age* (SHEFC, 2000). This is reflected in the current consultation on doctoral programmes being carried forward by the four UK higher education funding bodies (Metcalfe et al, 2002; HEFCE, 2003). Indeed, the inception of taught and professional doctorates was a fundamental driver in the impetus towards establishing quality and standards for programmes. Equally significant, and on a larger scale, is the project on re-envisioning the PhD in the USA. This project is a courageous attempt to engage all stakeholders in shaping the PhD for meeting the needs of the new millennium (Nyquist, 2002).

An issue of ongoing debate, both in respect of PhD and professional doctorate programmes, is the *amount* of coursework or teaching and learning (excluding supervision or mentorship) that is involved. As changes in the wider world impact upon academia, and as this has resulted in more organized approaches to PhD education, the differences between the two routes have sometimes become blurred. This is illustrated in Figure 1.1, which in a simplified way presents the situation within the UK. In some instances, while there has been a movement towards more coursework in some PhD programmes, there has been a drift within professional doctorates towards more emphasis on research. This trend creates a situation in which, in some UK higher education institutions, while there are often differences in the declared *goals* of the two routes, there is great difficulty in discerning any real variation in *content*. However, where such differences can be discerned, they emanate from the different intentions. While the emphasis in the PhD route is knowledge construction, the professional doctorate research element frequently incorporates a practice development

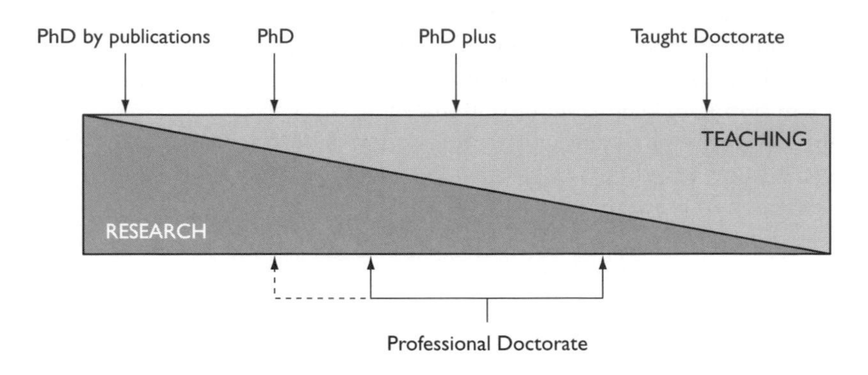

Figure 1.1 The UK teaching–research continuum

orientation. While in the former the emphasis is on advanced study in research methods, in the latter advanced professional studies are also usually included.

Conclusions

In this chapter we have attempted to address how the modern context and trends within it may impact upon the nature and content of doctoral preparation. As is often the case, we have succeeded only insofar as we have identified questions more than answers. However, this is how it should be. There is indeed a range of fundamental questions that the nursing profession must address. Paradoxically, these questions also relate to the future nature and content of doctoral education, while at the same time those in the ranks of postdoctoral nursing and those undertaking doctoral studies are those who must find answers to these questions. We do not have the answers to all the questions, but we have the basis for a dialogue within which they may be addressed. In one sense, this was the purpose of this chapter and indeed those that follow.

We might nevertheless identify some issues emerging from the current chapter that may contribute to the ongoing debate. We conclude by presenting these not as assertions that should necessarily be accepted or rejected, but rather as declarative statements that in the course of future dialogue should be challenged and indeed interrogated rigorously as we seek a way forward.

Declaration One: Confronting change The world is new, rapidly changing and increasingly global in its impact. We are called to review the nature of nursing, its professional orientation, and new ways of addressing new issues for which previous solutions are inadequate. This must reflect directly on the nature and content of doctoral education in nursing.

Declaration Two: Achieving clarity and consensus On an international level, while there are variations on the theme, doctoral education consists of a dichotomy between the PhD that primarily prepares researchers and other doctorates (of which the Professional Doctorate is the most common form) that aim to provide a wider preparation for research, leadership, education, managerial, advanced practice and/or practice development roles. There is a need for further clarity and consensus on this dichotomy, the differences in the two routes, or indeed the desirability of moving towards an acceptance of greater diversity in a range of routes.

Declaration Three: Widening dialogue In the past the issue of doctoral education, and indeed the role of postdoctoral nurses, has tended to be an issue largely restricted to the academic community. It must be assumed that those at the doctoral level within the profession have an important future role in establishing and enhancing the knowledge and practice base, and determining the future shape of the profession. Yet this issue has seldom been an important topic of debate within the wider profession, and at policy level such roles have often not been identified within human resources and strategic planning. Decisions in respect of the future nature, kind and content of doctoral education should be a matter for the profession as a whole. Leaders within the profession have a responsibility to ensure that such dialogue is carried forward, and that it is informed by and also informs healthcare policy. Importantly, we must also listen to the voices of those we serve, for they also must be involved in the shaping of the future of those who claim their best interests.

Declaration Four: Deciding content There is a broad consensus that doctoral education in whatever form should not be narrowly concerned with training in research skills. Nor should it be within a particular paradigm that is exclusively provided through mentorship/supervisory approaches, but should include other learning approaches and broader educational content that prepare doctoral candidates for postdoctoral professional life.

Declaration Five: Maintaining consistency and credibility While in general the aforementioned PhD/Professional Doctorate (or its equivalents) dichotomy may be helpful, as the issue of content of doctoral programmes is addressed, the range of programmes and diversity of content are increasing confusion within the profession as a whole and prospective doctoral candidates in particular. Although diversity is necessary for future development, there is a need to ensure that programmes have sufficient consistency at their core to have currency and credibility within the profession, within healthcare systems, and at national, international and global levels.

Declaration Six: Achieving balance On a global level, there is recognition, not only in nursing but also in other disciplines and across nations, that doctoral education is concerned with advancing knowledge and, in turn, practice. It is important that for the new millennium such preparation includes content that adequately prepares doctoral students for postdoctoral work in real-world situations. However, this should not compromise the universally accepted goal that such programmes prepare for research and scholarly inquiry. Although the ratio of what might be termed *research* to *supporting educational content* may vary between routes such as those identified in Declaration Two, careful attention must be given to the two aspects, how they are integrated and made complementary, and how appropriate balance is achieved.

Declaration Seven: Assuring quality It is recognized that quality assurance of education, including doctoral education, is increasingly emphasized at higher education institutional and national levels, and indeed in some instances is being addressed across nations. However, in an increasingly global context nursing has itself a vested interest in ensuring that doctoral education meets the demands of nursing for a sound knowledge and practice base across frontiers. The emerging global consciousness within nursing must be seen as an opportunity for working together, sharing best practices and developing doctoral education.

These declarative statements resonate through this book. The significant achievements and important advances in doctoral education must be readily acknowledged, and these are also well documented in the chapters that follow. Hopefully, here and in the remainder of this book we have demonstrated the current situation and the challenges to be met.

References

American Association of Colleges of Nursing (2001). *Indicators of quality in research-focused doctoral programs in nursing.* Washington, DC: AACN.

Argyris, C., and Schön, D. (1974). *Theory in practice: Increasing professional effectiveness.* London: Jossey-Bass.

Baker, M. E. (1998). Challenging ignorance. In: M. Baker and S. Kirk (eds). *Research and development for the NHS.* 2nd edn. Oxford: Radcliffe Medical Press.

Barrow, J. D. (1998). *Impossibility: The limits of science and the science of limits.* Oxford: Oxford University Press.

Beck, U. (1992). *Risk society: Towards a new modernity.* London: Sage.

Beck, U. (1997). *The reinvention of politics: Rethinking modernity in the global social order.* Cambridge: Polity Press.

Beck, U. (1999). *World risk society.* Malden, MA: Polity Press.

Beck, U. (2000). *What is globalization?* Malden, MA: Polity Press.

Beck, U. (2002). The silence of words and political dynamics in the World Risk Society. *Logos,* **1**(4). (http://logosonline.home.igc.org/beck.htm)

Benner, P. (1984). *From novice to expert: Excellence and power in clinical practice.* Menlo Park, CA: Addison Wesley.

Benner, P., Hooper-Kyriakidis, P. and Stannard, D. (1999). *Clinical wisdom and interventions in critical care: A thinking in action approach.* Philadelphia, PA: W. B. Saunders.

Bohm, D. (1980). *Wholeness and the implicate order.* New York, NY: Routledge, Chapman and Hall, Inc.

Bones, J. (Chair) (2002). *Professional doctorates.* Dudley: UK Council for Graduate Education (UKCGE).

Capra, F. (2002). *The hidden connections: A science for sustainable living.* London: Harper Collins.

Carpenter, D. R. and Hudacek, S. (1996). *On doctoral education in nursing: The voice of the student.* New York, NY: National League for Nursing Press.

Carr-Saunders, A. M. (1955). Metropolitan conditions and traditional professional relationships. In: A. M. Fisher (ed.). *The metropolis in modern life.* Garden City, NY: Rooksbury.

Davies, C. (1995). *Gender and the professional predicament in nursing.* Buckingham: Open University Press.

Deleuze, G. and Guattari, F. (1987). *A thousand plateaus. Capitalism and schizophrenia.* (Trans. B. Massumi). Minneapolis, MN: University of Minnesota Press.

Dickoff, J. and James, P. (1968). A theory of theories: A position paper. *Nursing Research*, **17**, 197–203.

European Ministers of Education (1999). *The Bologna Declaration: European Higher Education Area.* Joint Declaration of the European Ministers of Education convened in Bologna on 19 June 1999. Brussels: European Union.

Fawcett, J. (1984). The metaparadigm of nursing: Present status and future refinements. *Image: The Journal of Nursing Scholarship*, **16**, 84–87.

Fawcett, J. (2000). *Analysis and evaluation of contemporary nursing knowledge.* Philadelphia, PA: F. A. Davis.

Foucault, M. (1970). *The order of things: An archaeology of the human sciences.* London: Tavistock Publications Ltd.

Giddens, A. (1999). *Runaway world: How globalisation is reshaping our lives.* London: Profile.

Giddens, A. (2001). *The global third way debate.* Malden, MA: Polity Press.

Giddens, A. and Hutton, W. (2000). *On the edge: Living with global capitalism.* London: Jonathan Cape.

Henderson, V. (1966). *The nature of nursing: A definition and its implications for practice, research and education.* New York, NY: Macmillan.

Higher Education Funding Council for England, with Department for Employment and Learning, Northern Ireland, Higher Education Funding Council for Wales and Scottish Higher Education Funding Council (2003). *Improving standards in postgraduate research degree programmes: Formal consultation.* London: HEFCE.

Horgan, J. (1996). *The end of science: Facing the limits of knowledge in the twilight of the scientific age.* New York, NY: Addison Wesley.

Hugman, R. (1998). Social work and de-professionalisation. In: P. Abbott and L. Meerabeau (eds). *The sociology of the caring professions.* 2nd edn. London: UCL Press.

International Council of Nurses (1999). *Nurse retention, transfer, and migration.* Geneva: ICN.

Johnson, T. J. (1972). *Professions and power.* London: Macmillan.

Kuhn, T. (1970). *The structure of scientific revolutions.* Chicago, IL: University of Chicago Press.

Lunt, I. (2002). *Professional doctorates in education.* London: London University Institute of Education.

Lyotard, J-F. (1984). *The postmodern condition: A report on knowledge.* Manchester: Manchester University Press.

McKenna, H. and Cutcliffe, J. (2001). Nursing doctoral education in the United Kingdom and Ireland. *Online Journal of Issues in Nursing*, **5**, 2.

Magnet, J. (2003). What's wrong with nursing? *Prospect,* Issue 93, December 2003.
Metcalfe, J., Thompson, Q. and Green, H. (2002). *Improving standards in postgraduate research degree programmes: A report to the Higher Education Funding Councils of England, Scotland and Wales.* London: HEFCE.
Naisbitt, J. (1984). *Megatrends: Ten new directions transforming our lives.* London: Macdonald & Co.
Nyquist, J. D. (2002). The PhD: a tapestry of change for the 21st century. *Change,* **34**(6), 12–20.
Parry, N. and Parry, J. (1979). Social work, professionalism and the state. In: N. Parry, M. Rusten and C. Satyamurti (eds). *Social work, welfare and the state.* London: Edward Arnold.
Quality Assurance Agency for Higher Education (1999). *Code of practice for the assurance of academic quality and standards in higher education (postgraduate research programmes).* Gloucester, UK: QAA.
Said, E. (2000). *Reflections on exile and other essays.* Cambridge, MA: Harvard University Press.
Salvage, J. (1985). *The politics of nursing.* London: Heinemann Nursing.
Savage, J. (1987). *Nurses, gender and sexuality.* London: Heinemann Nursing.
Scottish Higher Education Funding Council (2000). *Research and the knowledge age.* Edinburgh: SHEFC.
Sergeant, H. (2003). *Managing not to manage.* London: Centre for Policy Studies.
Slevin, O. (1999). The nurse–patient relationship: Caring in a health context. In: A. Long (ed.). *Interaction for practice in community nursing.* London: Macmillan.
Slevin, O. (2003a). Nursing as a profession. In: L. Basford and O. Slevin (eds). *Theory and practice of nursing: An integrated approach to caring practice.* Cheltenham: Nelson Thornes.
Slevin, O. (Chair) (2003b). *Report of the initial review of the Doctor of Nursing Science (DNSc) programme.* Newtownabbey, Northern Ireland: University of Ulster.
Taylor, C. (1991). *The ethics of authenticity.* Cambridge, MA: Harvard University Press.
Toffler, A. (1970). *Future shock.* London: The Bodley Head.
Waldrop, M. M. (1992). *Complexity: The emergence of science at the edge of order and chaos.* New York, NY: Simon & Schuster.
Walsh, M. (2000). *Nursing frontiers: Accountability and the boundaries of care.* Oxford: Butterworth Heinemann.
Watson, J. (1990). Caring knowledge and informed moral passion. *Nursing Science Quarterly,* **13**(1), 15–24.
Watson, J. (1999). *Postmodern nursing and beyond.* Edinburgh: Churchill Livingstone.
World Health Assembly (1996). *Strengthening nursing and midwifery. Forty-ninth World Health Assembly – Resolution WHA 49.1.* Geneva: WHO.
World Health Assembly (2001). *Strengthening nursing and midwifery. Fifty-fourth World Health Assembly – Resolution WHA 54.12.* Geneva: WHO.

Chapter 2

Future directions in knowledge development and doctoral education in nursing

Ada Sue Hinshaw and Helena Leino-Kilpi

The knowledge base to guide nursing practice and healthcare has expanded dramatically in the past two decades in a number of regions of the world. As a critical mass of doctorally prepared nurses has built major research programmes focused on priority nursing and health problems in their countries, substantiated bodies of knowledge are evolving that enhance the quality of life for multiple populations and improve the healthcare provided to the public. This expansion of knowledge has been facilitated in a number of countries by nurse scientists' access to growing resources for conducting research. For example, Canadian nurse scholars are now highly successful competitors for federal research monies within most of the government's funding agencies for health and cancer research. In the Canadian health services research arena, there are targeted federal monies for nursing studies.

There is a symbiotic relationship between the expansion of knowledge in a discipline and its doctoral programmes; that is, as the cadre of doctorally prepared graduates grows, the research expands the knowledge base for the discipline and its practice, which in turn stimulates additional interest in doctoral education to acquire the competency and skills to further the science. Thus, the expansion of knowledge influences doctoral education while such education also impacts on the directions of knowledge development.

The development of knowledge through scientific inquiry is embedded in the context of the culture of the investigator's country (Ketefian and Redman, 1997). The research questions that are posed reflect the particular perspective and basic values of the investigator's cultural background. For example, in the USA, the nursing profession has a strong commitment to promoting the health of the public as well as ameliorating the consequences of illness. This orientation is evident in the research programmes developed by nurse scientists. The knowledge developed reflects the Western value for individualism and for promoting health through self-care and self-management behavioural strategies. In countries where infectious diseases are prominent in large populations there may be more focus on the immediate need to control the various illnesses.

Knowledge development within the nursing discipline is also greatly influenced by several factors within the country of the investigators. These factors include social issues, economic status, political events, demographic profiles of the populations and health/healthcare trends. For example, in a number of the countries with more developed economic and healthcare structures individuals are living longer. This has resulted in a growing cadre of older adults who are more prone to multiple chronic illnesses. These types of condition require increased care within the community rather than acute care settings, a situation that changes the pattern of delivery of healthcare (Callahan, 1985). In the USA, the PhD or Doctor of Philosophy degree is the culturally accepted preparation for research careers and is now being 're-envisioned' by many disciplines. The intent of the examination of this degree is to consider whether its orientation remains relevant given the numerous changes in the cultural, social and economic context of the country (Nyquist, 2002; see also Chapter 4).

The development of knowledge through the research programmes of nurse investigators will reflect both their cultural values and context as well as the current social, economic, political, demographic and health trends within their countries as stated above. In this chapter, two Western perspectives on building knowledge and developing doctoral programmes will be discussed and the major trends within the countries that shape the research questions and the evolving science will be considered. The two global regions/countries that will be examined are Europe, in particular Finland, and North America, in particular the USA.

Knowledge development and doctoral education: nursing scholarship in Europe and Finland

The continent of Europe has many countries. The European Union (EU, www.europa.eu.int; accessed on 18.8.2003), founded in 1993, is a union of 15 independent states. The EU was founded to enhance political, economic and social cooperation between the countries of Europe. Finland joined the EU in 1995, and at present the other members are: Austria, Belgium, Denmark, France, Germany, Greece, Ireland, Italy, Luxembourg, the Netherlands, Portugal, Spain, Sweden and United Kingdom of Great Britain and Northern Ireland (UK). Ten more countries joined the European Union in 2004: Cyprus (Greek section), the Czech Republic, Estonia, Hungary, Latvia, Lithuania, Malta, Poland, Slovakia and Slovenia.

The educational context for doctoral education in nursing in the EU includes the growth of education generally, research and development of the countries and the emerging issues for doctoral education. During the course of the 1990s the number of people in tertiary level education increased. In the EU, 16% of people over 15 years of age go for third level education (Strack, 2003; www.europa.eu.int/ comm/eurostat; accessed 17.8.2003). In proportion to the population, Finland has the highest number of people who have third level education – by 2001, nearly a quarter of people aged 15 and over. This is more than 50% higher than the average in the rest of the EU.

In 2002, the countries of the EU agreed the target of raising research and development (R&D) investment to 3% of the gross national product (GDP) by the year 2010. The aim was to make the EU, by 2010, the most competitive and dynamic knowledge-based economy in the world. At the time of writing, only Finland and Sweden have exceeded the 3% target level (Academy of Finland, 2003).

Doctoral degrees have been an essential part of higher education in Europe for over eight centuries. In 1987, the Organisation for Economic Cooperation and Development (OECD) (Noble, 1994; Blume, 1995) identified the emerging problems of growing postgraduate education, drawing attention to the long duration of postgraduate studies. In the 1990s, the OECD (1991, 1995) recommended that postdoctoral positions should be increased, and graduate school model should be implemented. At present, there still is a need for developing more systematic information on European postgraduate education (Frijdal and Bartelse, 1999).

Nursing research in Europe

In Europe, the history of nursing research goes back to 1950, starting in the UK (Tierney, 1997). In the Nordic countries, nursing research has been progressing since the end of 1960s (Hamrin, 1990; Lauri, 1990; Lerheim, 1990; Lorensen, 1990). The Nordic Academy of Nursing Science (NASV) was established in 1991. On a European level, the Workgroup of European Nurse Researchers (WENR, 1997, www.wenr.org; accessed 18.8.2003) was established in 1978 with the aim of building contacts between nurse researchers; this organization includes 25 European national nurses' associations. It collects yearly information about nursing and nursing research in member countries. In addition, the World Health Organization (WHO) Regional Office for Europe, the International Council of Nurses (ICN), and the International Council of Midwives launched a Europe-wide 'Health21 Campaign' aimed at strengthening the health impact of nurses and midwifes (WHO, 1999).

In 1996, the Council of Europe made five recommendations for nursing research in Europe. The recommendations proposed to develop: (i) the structure and organization for nursing research; (ii) the integration of research and practice; (iii) education for nursing research; (iv) funding for nursing research; and (v) national and international collaboration. A year later, WENR (1997) surveyed the impact of the recommendations. Feedback was positive, but real impact was not so clear, especially on the governmental level. Nevertheless, these Europe-wide recommendations became a landmark in the European history of nursing research. More recently, WENR (2003) published a Position Paper on nursing research in Europe. In this paper, WENR recommends that nursing research take into account the following: clinical outcomes, multidisciplinary work between all health and social care professionals and evidence-based practice.

All these documents and recommendations indicate the importance of nursing research in Europe. In some countries, these recommendations have already been realized. In some countries, they are being used politically to try to get support for the establishment of academic nursing education. In the Nordic countries a symposium was held in 1995, about priorities in nursing/caring science (Hamrin and Lorensen, 1997). Some general recommendations for the future were made: promotion of health and wellbeing across the life-span of an individual, symptom management, care of the elderly, cost-effectiveness evaluation, restructuring healthcare systems, self-management of health and illness, and development of knowledge from theoretical/philosophical perspectives.

In 2001, in a symposium about knowledge development in nursing/caring arranged by NASV, nursing science was analysed from the perspective of philosophy, ethics, social sciences, humanistic sciences and natural sciences. Based on the analysis, researchers in the Nordic countries were committed to the importance of nursing/caring sciences, and noted the high degree of multidisciplinary collaboration and strong interest for doctoral studies. More meta-analytic studies, concept analysis and theoretical studies were recommended.

In Finland, the Nursing Research Institute was established in 1966 and academic master's and doctoral level education started in 1979 (Sinkkonen, 1988; Lauri, 1990). A review of licentiate and doctoral studies (Leino-Kilpi and Suominen, 1998; Suominen and Leino-Kilpi, 1998), and articles published in the *Finnish Yearbook of Nursing* and in the *Journal of Nursing Science* from 1958 to 1995, pointed out that most of the research at that time was descriptive in nature with emphasis on quantitative methods and concentrated on the practice of nursing and primary healthcare. There was a lack of methodologic research and concept analysis. This was also the case in Sweden (e.g. Segersten, 1993). International collaboration was challenged.

Today, nursing research has a strong position in Finnish society as part of health sciences. Research priorities (e.g. Eriksson, 1997; Hoitotiede-lehti, 1999; Academy of Finland, 2000) in the universities include theory construction, nursing philosophy and ethics, preventive nursing, family nursing, clinical nursing with different foci and also nursing education and health management science. Finnish researchers actively publish in international journals; for example, during 1997–2001 they collectively published more than 400 articles.

There is a national strategy for nursing and nursing research in Finland (Perälä, 1998). Several recommendations are included in this strategy such as a stronger role for nursing research, closer connections between research and practice, focusing the research on important areas of Finnish health policy, emphasis on the development of research skills, systematic funding for research and development of evaluative systems. In 2003 the Academy of Finland started an international evaluation of Finnish nursing research and the results of the evaluation will provide some recommendations for the future.

Recently, Evers (2003) described the developing nursing science in Europe. He emphasized the empirical nature of nursing science and the importance of clinically relevant problems related to nursing needs or nursing diagnosis of the people of Europe. According to him, nurse researchers must combine theory and empirical evidence – and disseminate scientific nursing knowledge widely both to the public and to nurses themselves. The need for evidence-based nursing has been pointed out by many other authors in Europe as well. Evidence-based nursing is still at an early stage of development, although it is growing steadily in many countries (WHO, 2002; Elomaa, 2003).

Doctoral nursing education in Europe

Academic education in nursing in Europe at the university level was first established in the UK in 1950s (Hamrin, 1997; McKenna and Cutcliffe, 2001). Today, academic nursing education is the norm in most of the member states of the EU, and much progress is ongoing (van Maanen, 1998 www.wenr.org, www.ocenf.org, accessed 18.8.2003). In Finland (Leino-Kilpi and Uski, 2001), programmes for doctoral degrees exist in five universities: Kuopio, Oulu, Tampere, Turku and Abo Akademi (in Swedish). In these universities, most of the faculty are PhD-prepared.

In the 1990s, there was an increase in the numbers of nurses holding doctoral degrees in many countries. In 1992, there were about 160 nurses with doctorates in Sweden, 40 in Finland, 13 in Denmark, 20 in Norway and 7–8 in Iceland (Hamrin, 1997). In Finland, the number of doctorates has been rapidly increasing. The first doctoral graduation took place in 1984, and today, there are close to 200 doctorally prepared nurses. Between 1997 and 2002 there were 118 graduates and numbers are increasing: in 1997, there were 11 PhD-graduates from the five universities and in 2001 the corresponding number was 24. The same growth trend is seen in other disciplines in Finland (Academy of Finland, 2003). Despite these advances, there are relatively small numbers of doctorally prepared nurses in the European region.

The type of doctorate available for nurses is usually the PhD, as is the case in other Nordic countries. There are two ways to conduct doctoral study (Hamrin, 1997; Rahm-Hallberg, 2003): as a monograph prepared at the end of doctoral studies or as a composite dissertation including internationally published papers and a summary. The latter has a stronger tradition in the universities where academic nursing education takes place in the medical faculties, as is the case with three Finnish universities (Oulu, Tampere and Turku). The doctoral student chooses the way to present the study, but it also depends on the topic: there are more international opportunities to publish in clinical fields, than, for example, in nursing education. Also, the selection is dependent on the linguistic skills of the doctoral students.

The field of study for doctoral students depends on the research programme of the university. In Finland, clinically oriented dissertations are most common, followed by those in nursing education and administration. This seems to be the common trend in the other Nordic countries, too. Research programmes in universities are more or less homogeneous, and the content is dependent on the health and nursing priorities in the country. One of the main problems in many countries is that there are too few nursing professors and other senior researchers for the supervision of doctoral students. Senior researchers, thus, have more than one area to study but even then many important fields of nursing remain without any funded research projects.

In Finland, the Ministry of Education established the graduate school system in 1995. Within the next few years the Government of Finland made the important decision to increase public funding for this system. In nursing science, there is also a National Doctoral School with ten enrolled doctoral students who are also employed. This national school is working in collaboration with the five universities. The universities organize four to five national doctoral courses together annually, invite international researchers and support the networking of doctoral students. Based on the report of the Ministry of Education (2000), there has been a gradual decrease in the number of years to completion of the doctoral dissertation, and about 60% of students completed their doctoral studies within the prescribed four years of study. The mean age of nursing science PhD students (40 years) is high compared with other disciplines (median for all disciplines was 36 years in 1999), but there is a decreasing trend at the National Doctoral School. Graduation at a later age means less time to establish a research career and this, in turn, inhibits the systematic development of knowledge in the field.

Influence of demographic, social and political factors, and health priorities on nursing research and doctoral education

Ageing population

In 1999, the population of the EU was about 375 million people. A main demographic factor influencing the need for doctoral nursing education is the ageing of the population. Ageing means an increasing proportion of elderly people in the population and, individually, it means increasing life expectancy. According to the OECD *Health Data* (www.oecd.fr; accessed 15.8.2003) in Finland, for example, life expectancy has increased by about 10 years since the 1960s and the trend is similar in most of the member states of EU (www.europa.eu.int/comm/eurostat; accessed 17.8.2003; European Commission, 2003). In 1990, the average of the old-age dependency ratio (ratio of older people to people in traditional working age) in the OECD countries was 19% (Hicks, 1996). By 2030, this could nearly double to 37%. The growth will be particularly rapid after 2010 in the population over 80 years of age.

Ageing is an individual process. It means that the number of people of retirement age is growing and they need more health services. This situation has financial ramifications, and requires new patterns of care-giving to families. The elderly population is also living rather well: based on the study among nine OECD countries (OECD, 2001) older people at all income levels tend to maintain their material standards of living once they stop working. This happens despite differences in approaches to public policy, such as pensions.

Nurses take care of elderly people in their homes, communities, primary healthcare settings, hospitals, long-term institutions and nursing homes. In nursing education, there are programmes for elderly nursing, and this is one of the main foci of nursing research. In Finland, the Academy of Finland has funded a large national multidisciplinary research programme in ageing and development of health services for the elderly population. Nurse researchers have developed theories for nursing care of elderly people in homes and long-term facilities. In these research groups, doctoral students have a major role. A need for a nationwide nursing research project in elderly nursing care, in which doctoral students could be immersed and mentored, has been identified as a priority for the future.

Health priorities

Health priorities are dependent on many factors. Current available data do not allow the systematic measurement of health status in a way that does justice to the concept by including measures of quality of life – a concept more close to nursing. Statistics usually look at causes of death, morbidity, and disability. In Finland, for example, the main causes of death are cardiovascular diseases, cancer, pneumonia and other infections, cerebrovascular diseases and accidents (Aromaa, 1994; www.who.int; accessed 19.8.2003). Infant mortality is one of the lowest in the world (OECD, 2003). These data are very similar in Nordic countries (European Commission, 2003): cardiovascular disease is the main cause of death in women in all countries of Europe and is the main cause of death in men in all countries except France.

In Europe, women (15 years and older) enjoy a high level of health as measured by a variety of health indicators (www.europa.eu.int/comm/health). Life expectancy has increased, maternal mortality is low, women perceive themselves as healthy and have been getting taller. In spite of this generally good health status, there are problems with disability, activity limitations, mental disorders and accidents. Special issues in women's health are eating disorders, human immunodeficiency virus/acquired immune deficiency syndrome, osteoporosis, as well as violence against women.

The vast majority of young people in Europe enjoy good health (European Commission, 2000). There are, however, also many specific health issues. Among these are inequalities in young people's health between families, population subgroups and countries, substance abuse and mental disorders. In Finland, for example, within the past few years, more resources in healthcare have been geared to mental health of children and adolescents.

Globally, the major health risks have been analysed by the WHO (www.who.int; accessed 19.8.2003). This analysis points out risks as follows: childhood and maternal under-nutrition, diet-related risks, physical inactivity, sexual and reproductive health, addictive substances, environmental risks and occupational risks. Only some of these issues are relevant to Finland, Nordic countries or Europe. For example, physical inactivity is a risk for many health problems, like cardiovascular diseases, high blood pressure and overweight. Risk factors in the area of sexual and reproductive health can affect wellbeing in a number of ways. The largest risk by far is that posed by unsafe sex leading to infection with HIV/AIDS. The numbers of these infections are still low in Finland and Nordic countries, but they are increasing. Also, the same increasing trend can be identified for addictive substances (OECD, 2003). Environmental and occupational risks are partly related to each other. In the Nordic countries, these are manifested in environmental problems in urban areas, as work-related carcinogens, and ergonomic and psychological stressors.

What does the analysis of health risks mean to doctoral education in nursing? It means that nursing research needs to respond to these health issues and risk factors in many countries, if not globally. However, there is not much research collaboration globally, or between the major world regions. There are, however, numerous international research projects within Europe, between and among European, US and Canadian universities; more recently, research collaboration has included researchers from Australia, Japan and Taiwan as well. These efforts should be fostered in the future. The health risks described mean that there is still a need for nursing research in the areas of prevention, health education, healthy ways of living, health impact assessments and evaluation of the outcomes of health promotion. In the Nordic countries, there is an emphasis on health promotion in health policies, maternity care, care of children and school healthcare. In spite of this emphasis, however, there is a need for evaluation of health promotion. It is especially the case that cardiovascular and long-term diseases require research. It is critical therefore that doctoral students learn to analyse the health risks, and be able to use the information included in the health statistics in their projects.

Social and economic factors

The major determinants of health problems are behavioural (e.g. smoking, lack of physical activity, drug addiction), poor environmental conditions and low socio-economic status (European Commission, 2003 www.who.int; accessed 19.8.2003). The vast majority of threats to health are more commonly found among poor people, people with little formal education, and those with lowly occupations. One in eight people lived in a jobless household in the EU in 1999, but there are major differences between the countries (Eurostat, 2003a, 2003b). Looking at the monetary indicators, at-risk-of-poverty rate is highest in Portugal and Greece, and lowest in Sweden, Finland, the Netherlands, Denmark and Germany.

Economic factors include, among others, the total expenditure on health in the country (% gross domestic product (GPD), OECD, 2003). In Finland, this has increased from 5.6% in 1970s to 7% in 2001. The corresponding percentages in the USA are higher: 6.9% and 13.9% respectively. Per capita expenditure in 2001 for Finland was US$1841, and for the USA US$4887. The variation, of course, reflects the differences in healthcare systems. It also informs us on how health is valued in the social policy of the country.

Economic factors can be identified both at a macro level (e.g. GPD per capita) and at an individual micro level, and they depend on the system of social security and healthcare policy in the countries. In the Nordic countries, earnings are most equitably distributed, individual living standards are good and the level of education is high. The greatest inequalities in Europe seem to occur in Spain and the UK (European Commission, 2003). Nursing research has focused on individual poverty rather than community level political decisions in resource allocation. In future, both of these levels should receive attention in nursing research. This is a useful field for multidisciplinary research projects.

Women's lives have changed in Europe during the past three decades (www.europa.eu.int/comm/health; accessed 30.7.2003). The rate of marriage has declined and the average age at first marriage (26.1 years) and at first birth (28.6 years) have risen. Women's participation in the labour force has increased (there are variations across Europe). The Nordic countries have the highest rates of gender equality, in part because of higher levels of education and income relative to men.

Nursing research is concerned with families, communities and their healthcare. Traditionally, the family represents the first source of informal healthcare and the major support system for the young and the old. Thus, family structures are important sources of companionship and are associated with patterns of mental health, as well as other health problems. This means that all areas of family nursing are of great importance for doctoral study, and this is further emphasized because of ageing populations and shorter lengths of hospitalization.

Healthcare organization

Healthcare organization, healthcare personnel and the needs of nursing workforce are also related to doctoral nursing education. 1998 estimates of health personnel in European countries vary among nurses: In Greece there are 257 nurses/100,000 population; the corresponding number in Finland is 2162 and in the USA 972 (www.who.int; accessed 19.8.2003). Adding to this, the nursing workforce profile (ICN, 2003) gives interesting information. For example, the average age of employed nurses varies between 30 years in Germany and 44.7 years in Sweden; in USA it is 43.3 years. This means that there will be many retirements in the future. The employment status also varies. In Iceland, for example, nurses employed full time (35 hours or more/week) comprise 25% of the total nursing population, with 43% in Norway, 49% in Denmark, 55% in Sweden and 72% in the USA.

The healthcare systems in the Nordic countries have many similarities. For example, the principal employer in the Nordic countries is the public sector. Since the 1990s, there have been many changes in the healthcare organizations. These have to do with acute care: number of beds and average length of stay in hospital have decreased (OECD, 2003). Finland illustrates this change: in the 1960s the average length of stay in acute care was 12.5 days, in 2001 it dropped to 4.4 days. In the USA, it was 7.6 days in the 1960s and 5.8 days now, which does not indicate as large a change as in the Nordic countries.

In many countries, the challenges for their healthcare systems are similar. The European Observatory on Health Care Systems (2002) conducted an analysis of eight countries in Europe including Denmark, France, Germany, the Netherlands, Sweden and the UK. Major challenges in these countries had to do with cost management, ageing, quality programmes, limited resources, long waiting lists for patients, shortage of medical and nursing staff, issues in public healthcare and community, and also questions about the realization of patients' rights.

For nurse researchers, changes in organization are also a challenge. Nurses' roles, particularly in nursing-sensitive outcomes, are of great importance. Also, the role of patients has changed: the shorter stay in hospitals and increasing numbers of day-surgeries, increasing nursing responsibility for teaching and supervising patients, and increasing need for home care nursing and community support. In the nursing knowledge base, empowerment of patients is important. We still do not know enough about the empowering process and the role of nurses in that process.

Patients' rights are part of the ethical knowledge base in nursing. Rights include, for example, the right to access medical treatment and nursing care, the right to information and the right to high level, professional care. In Finland, these are defined in the Act on Patients' Status and Rights (No 785/1992, www.finlex.fi; accessed 15.7.2003). To date, ethics has not been in the mainstream of nursing research. The situation changed somewhat in Europe in the 1990s, because of the research funding by the European Commission. For example, funding has been provided for nursing research in the areas of autonomy, privacy, and informed consent of patients in elderly care, postnatal and surgery nursing (e.g. Leino-Kilpi et al, 2000) and for research in ethical codes in nursing (www.ecn.nl; accessed 15.7.2003). Doctoral students from many European countries have been involved in these initiatives.

Information and communication technologies are economic factors in healthcare organization. Investment in information and communication technology has been the most dynamic component in recent years (OECD, 2002), technology has been developed in hospitals, primary healthcare and for improving communication between people's homes and the healthcare organization. Communications equipment was the most important area for investment in

2000 in Finland; the highly skilled information and communication technology workers had an annual growth rate of about 49% during 1997–1999. This means that new technology has been invested in nursing as well, giving rise to the need to study the outcomes of such technology.

Doctoral students in nursing science are mostly experienced nurses within the Nordic countries. Experience supports understanding of issues in healthcare organization from different perspectives. Experience also produces relevant research questions about healthcare organizations and understanding to formulate projects in that field. In summary, evaluation of healthcare organization is deemed an appropriate area for research for doctoral students in nursing.

Future challenges for doctoral education in Europe

Despite the growth described earlier, there are still a limited number of doctorally prepared nurses in Europe. On the one hand there are still countries without any academic nursing education and on the other there are many countries with high level academic education and research – and there is increasing collaboration between countries. Inside the EU, for example, the Socrates and Erasmus exchange programmes have provided opportunities for doctoral nursing students to create international networks. Collaboration also takes place through the European Academy for Nursing (EANS, www.eans.org; accessed 20.7.2003), the Nordic Academy for Advanced Study (Norfa) and different agreements between European universities. The Nordic countries support nurse researchers in the Baltic countries. Also, in many countries there is national collaboration between universities. In addition, more funding is available through the European Commission, new scientific journals have been established, and the numbers of presentations at conferences and publications have increased. All these developments enhance new ideas for knowledge development and doctoral education.

There are many challenges in knowledge development and doctoral education in nursing for the future.

1. Nursing research should reflect the health problems in the country or relevant region. This requires doctoral students to analyse the health issues in their country and produce relevant knowledge for supporting nurses working with clients. Based on the health statistics, in Europe there is a need to study, in particular, patients with cardiac diseases, cancer and chronic illnesses (Jonsdottir, 2001), as well as issues connected with healthy ways of living and health promotion. There is also a need to study mental health problems, problems caused by changes in health organization, family nursing issues (Tomlinson and Hall, 2003) and disease prevention. The ethical knowledge base should be strengthened.
2. The need for evidence-based nursing is recommended for doctoral students.

This challenge is mainly methodological: they need to be educated in experimental designs.

3 Doctoral students need to be educated in the field of health problems of ageing populations. Health issues today are more complicated because of the ageing population and new technologies in medicine. To be able to approach these issues, doctoral students in nursing need to work and learn in multidisciplinary research teams. Such teams should include medical and other health science students (Rahm-Hallberg, 2003).
4 Universities need to have an active interchange with the community; in nursing this means active collaboration between researchers, doctoral students and nurses in practice. In Finland this has been supported by establishing a cross-appointment position for professors between universities and university hospitals in each of the five universities.
5 Nursing research is not only concerned with health issues and supporting nursing problems in practice. Doctoral students need to participate in theory construction, instrument development and philosophical analysis of science. Without this, nursing does not meet the requirements of an academic discipline.
6 International collaboration between nurse researchers is a fact today, at least in many European countries. International collaboration often means empirical data collection in more than one country. Data collection implies different research ethical issues and learning experiences, as indicated by the Working Group for the Study of Ethical Issues in International Nursing Research (2003).
7 There is a need to study the outcomes of health information and communication technologies, both in hospitals and communities. By using technology effectively, some problems of nursing shortages could be solved.
8 A very limited number of universities offer postdoctoral education. Researchers are encouraged to find colleagues interested in the same health and nursing issues to work with. Presently, it seems to be relatively easy for doctoral students to find international partners. This is the case particularly among those students who make a composite dissertation and publish papers from their studies during doctoral education.

Knowledge development and doctoral education: nursing scholarship in North America

For both the North American countries (Canada and the USA), the expanding body of knowledge reflects the values of the countries and more specifically, the nursing discipline's strong focus on the health of individuals, their families, as well as communities. There is a commitment to promoting health as well as facilitating individual response to illness and disease conditions. The emphasis is on the whole individual, family or community rather than on the illness or disease (Stewart, 1997; Hébert, 2003). In both countries, the attention of the investigators in the scientific community has been on generating clinical nursing research programmes and programmes focused on shaping the environment for nursing practice. In Canada, a number of clinical research programmes have focused on palliative care for individuals and families experiencing end-of-life concerns, understanding and managing chronic illness, health promotion, and issues in women's health (ACEN et al, 2002). The same types of issues are identified in the first *Handbook of Clinical Nursing Research* published in the USA (Hinshaw et al, 1999). The doctoral programmes in both countries reflect seminars and concentrations focused on these areas of clinical nursing research. In addition, doctoral education in the two countries includes many core courses on theory development, research methodologies, measurement strategies and statistical processes. From a methodological perspective, the holistic philosophical commitment has demanded a pluralistic approach. Qualitative and quantitative methods are both valued for the richness they provide to the research data.

In North America, the development of knowledge through research has increased rapidly due to expanding resources. With the establishment of the National Institute of Nursing Research (NINR) at the National Institutes of Health (NIH) in 1986 (Merritt, 1986) nursing research in the USA advanced dramatically. Starting with slightly over US$11 million for research and research training in 1986 to over US$130 million in 2003, strong support has been provided for the generation of knowledge for nursing practice and research training monies for institutional grants and individual fellowships for doctoral and postdoctoral education.

Three major Canadian organizations, the Academy of Canadian Executive Nurses (ACEN), the Association of Canadian Academic Healthcare Organizations (ACAHO), and the Canadian Association of University Schools of Nursing (CAUSN) identified the four primary federal and private funding agencies for nursing research: Canadian Institutes of Health Research (CIHR), Canadian Health Services Research Foundation (CHSRF), the Canadian Foundation for Innovation (CFI) and the Social Science Health Research Council (SSHRC) (ACEN et al, 2002). While there is no designated funding agency for nursing research, Canadian nurse scholars are quite active and successful in competing for research and research training funds. In some areas, such as research training, specific monies are allocated for 'capacity building in nursing research'. In 2001 and 2002, CASN reported that nursing research funding from all sources totaled CAN$31,843,905 and CAN$17,872,567, respectively. In the new CIHR, established in 2000, Canadian scholars are active members of seven of the 13 institute advisory boards and are competing for research funding in several of the new institutes.

As in the USA, the expansion of resources has advanced the clinical research and health services nursing research programmes. But in both countries, there is room for far more growth, first in the area of resources, and second, in the research and research training programmes. The current expansion of knowledge for nursing has increased the opportunities for doctoral education.

Contextual factors influencing knowledge development/doctoral programmes

The development of knowledge to guide nursing practice in Canada and the USA has been influenced by multiple social, economic, political, demographic and healthcare contextual factors. In turn, these factors have shaped doctoral education in the nursing discipline in both countries.

Social factors influencing knowledge development and doctoral programmes

From a social perspective, a major concern in the USA and Canada is the disparity in healthcare including access to and the quality of health care, as well as outcomes for patients and their families. A recent Institute of Medicine (IOM) report (2003a), *Unequal treatment: confronting racial and ethnic disparities in health care,* reviewed several studies confirming the existence of disparity in relation to race, ethnicity and socioeconomic position, e.g. those who are uninsured for healthcare in the USA. These factors affect the healthcare people receive and subsequently their health (Waidmann and Rajan, 2000; Villarruel, 2001). Research shows that the incidence of certain diseases as well as the morbidity and mortality outcomes for several conditions such as cardiovascular disease, premature infants and cancer treatment differ among individuals of minority populations and between men and women (Sternberg, 2001). It is becoming increasingly evident that part of the difficulty is the disparity in people's access to healthcare and differences in the diagnosis and treatment processes (Jackson et al, 2002).

A series of reports by the IOM on the large population of uninsured people in the USA suggests that such individuals seek healthcare late in an illness trajectory, experience more complications and incur higher economic costs to themselves and society (IOM, 2002). Losing or not having health insurance impacts on families and total communities, not just individuals. The most recent report, *A Shared Destiny*, outlines how the 'quality, quantity, and scope' of health services within a community are influenced by a sizeable uninsured population (IOM, 2003b).

Even with the Canadian health system of care for all citizens, the particular needs of vulnerable populations are still of concern. Inequalities still exist in the healthcare system (Browne et al, 2001). Inequities also occur in healthcare research with issues of women's health not always being well attended. Many nurse researchers are delighted with the new Institute of Gender and Health which is part of the CIHR established in 2000 (Stewart et al, 2001) as a forum for addressing concerns about the differences in health issues between men and women.

Health disparities (USA) or inequalities (Canada) have surfaced as a strong priority for nursing research given the profession's commitment to vulnerable populations (Butler et al, 2002). Specifically, the approach focuses on identifying the areas in which disparities occur and preventing these situations. Nurse investigators in both countries have developed centres for studying health disparities, particularly in minority populations and are developing the knowledge needed to counter such problems. The doctoral and master's programmes are incorporating health disparities and inequalities in the curriculums and providing doctoral students opportunities to study such issues with the faculty funded for health disparities research (Villarruel, 2001).

Economic factors influencing knowledge development and doctoral programmes

The cost of healthcare in the USA is escalating rapidly. Major steps have been taken to contain and curtail such costs. The acute care hospitals have been the prime focus of new healthcare cost models since they provide the majority of the care and have been so expensive. A number of managed care models have been developed with a common purpose: to control costs and improve quality and access to healthcare. By 1995, over 60% of the total US population belonged to some type of managed care (IOM, 1997b). One of the major strategies for controlling costs was to shift as much of the healthcare as possible to community agencies. This shift to community care was accompanied by a strong philosophical approach focused on self-care or self-management by individuals and families of their healthcare issues. With nursing's long history of working in the community, their services were in high demand through home care, community public health and hospice agencies.

Major research programmes of nurse scientists in the USA and Canada have focused on chronic illnesses, primarily care in the community and health promotion, risk reduction and self-management studies. Prevention and self-management of chronic illness are perceived as cost containment strategies for healthcare. Concentrations in both of these areas have been developed in many of the nursing doctoral programmes in both countries. A number of centres of excellence that have been established in schools of nursing in the USA focused on, for example, health promotion across the life span or health promotion among the elderly population. Stewart (1997) outlined the Canadian commitment to health promotion describing the 14 centres launched in this area in the past ten years. These centres provide doctoral students with the experience of being immersed in these areas of research if that is their interest.

Another major economic factor that has influenced the development of knowledge for nursing practice in the USA was the doubling of the NIH budget and concurrently, doubling of the NINR budget. The NINR is the major funding body for nursing research in the USA. The commitment to health research on the part of the public and the Congress of the USA, and their determination to double the NIH budget in order to stimulate more research has greatly increased knowledge development for nursing. The funding for nursing research grants went from 56 million in1998 to over 130 million in 2003 (Grady, 2003). This higher level of funding for nurse investigators has also provided enhanced opportunities for doctoral students to work with their study teams and to do research. In addition, the research training funds to support doctoral students and postdoctoral fellows also doubled from 4.6 million in 1998 to 9.3 million in 2002, increasing the numbers of individuals in full-time study.

In Canada, the federal agency for funding health research – CIHR – was established in 2000. This replaces the old Medical Research Council. Nurse investigators and leaders expect to have increased access to shaping the nation's policies and acquiring funding from the CIHR. Nurse researchers have been active members of the Governing Council, sit on seven of the 13 institute advisory boards, and a number of the research review committees. According to Alcock (2002) nurse investigators' success rate in acquiring funding from CIHR is increasing, but greater growth can be achieved.

Political factors influencing knowledge development and doctoral programmes

The major political influence on knowledge development in the health sciences in the USA is the terrorist event of 11 September 2001 that destroyed the World Trade Center in New York City and killed many individuals. The USA reacted to the event as a 'wake-up' call for any number of terrorist events that could occur. Obviously, in the health field, biological, chemical, radiological and other such events are being considered. This response has led to multiple centres for bioterrorism and preparedness for bioterrorism being established in universities across the country. However, terrorism and bioterrorism are not confined to one country given the long, common border between Canada and the USA. This has provided new fields of study and new opportunities for doctoral students to be involved in funded research.

Demographic factors influencing knowledge development and doctoral programmes

In Canada and the USA, the fastest growing population is the cohort of individuals over 85 years (Algase, 2001). The number of individuals 65 years of age and over is rapidly increasing. These demographics raise several important issues for nursing and the knowledge for nursing practice. One issue is the high number of individuals and families experiencing chronic illnesses in the over-65 population, as discussed earlier. In addition, the issues involved with families and care-giving responsibilities are critical – issues that nurses are intimately involved in while caring for families. Another concern is the 'approaching death' issue (IOM, 1997a), of increasing concern to individuals and families who are involved with end-of-life decisions. These are all issues that nurse investigators are studying. A number of doctoral programmes offer concentrations in end-of-life, palliative care, family care-giving and chronic illness adaptation, as knowledge is rapidly evolving with the faculty building strong research programmes in these fields. Doctoral students are offered research experiences in such investigative programmes in both countries (Callahan, 1985; ACEN et al, 2002).

Health trends influencing knowledge development and doctoral programmes

Several health trends have influenced knowledge development for nursing practice. The genetic revolution is rapidly changing the practice of medicine and nursing as well as other health professions. Treatment therapies, symptom management, and family counselling are only a few of the areas that are dramatically affected by the exploding knowledge in genetics. The knowledge of genetics will revolutionize nursing practice and research globally. The research programmes of nurse investigators have only just begun to illustrate the major changes that will be demanded in nursing practice. A limited number of doctoral programmes are beginning to offer concentrations and research experiences in nursing with a genetic component.

In the USA, another healthcare trend has been the restructuring of acute care hospitals due to managed care and the need to control costs. Strategies for controlling costs resulted in the creation of hospital environments that were not conducive to adequate staffing and quality nursing practice. Research shows that poor patient outcomes and higher mortality accompanied inadequate staffing (Buerhaus, 2000; Aiken et al, 2003). In the nursing systems areas, knowledge is being developed regarding adequate staffing levels for nursing and the development of environments to facilitate better patient outcomes, as well as the recruitment and retention of nurses in healthcare facilities (McClure and Hinshaw, 2002). Thus, doctoral nursing students interested in creating stronger environments for professional practice and quality patient outcomes, can select programmes with faculty conducting research in nursing and organizational systems (IOM, 2003c). In Canada, research has also focused on human resources and health systems. The health systems differ greatly between the two countries but there are similar resource issues with the shortage of nurses and how to shape efficient work environments to recruit and retain nurses who can provide quality nursing care (O'Brien-Pallas et al, 2002).

In summary, a number of contextual factors influencing knowledge development in the nursing discipline and doctoral programmes have been considered. Examples of the major aspects of each factor, particularly as it impacts on doctoral education and knowledge evolution in nursing have been provided.

Priorities for knowledge development: future directions for doctoral programmes

Knowledge development in the USA and Canada has advanced from broad concepts with limited research substantiation to the refinement of concepts and testing of the relationships among them. Many research programmes for nurse investigators provide evidence for the development of the concepts and relationships (Hinshaw et al, 1999; Hébert, 2003). Knowledge development in the discipline has consistently focused on knowledge for a purpose; i.e. to guide nursing practice. The evolving knowledge base is built from a nursing perspective to provide evidence for the practice of the profession. The knowledge will be used by and built on by many investigators in numerous disciplines but for the purpose of nursing, it focuses on critical healthcare issues that nurses can influence through their practice, and thus 'make a difference' in the quality of life and health of the nations' people.

Concurrent with the advancement of the knowledge base for nursing, there have been changes in the doctoral programmes. In the early stage of knowledge development (mid-1970s), the majority of the courses offered in the doctoral curricula were process-oriented in nature, dealing with theory construction, research methodologies and statistical analysis. While these types of courses continue to be offered, doctoral programmes now provide multiple areas of content concentration reflecting the refinement of science: e.g. palliative care, women's health, family care and the frail elderly, health promotion behavioural change strategies, and bio-behavioral interventions for symptom management.

Numerous priorities have shaped the directions of nursing research. Usually, the priorities reflect the critical health and illness issues of the country. In 2000, four major priorities were reported for six or more countries/regions (Africa, European Nursing Research Work Group, Great Britain, the Nordic countries, Thailand, and the USA): health promotion, care of the elderly, health care systems and symptom management (Hinshaw, 2000). The USA was one of the five countries citing the need for these four areas of study. These priorities are already evident in the content offered by a number of US and Canadian doctoral programmes.

In the USA, the NINR facilitated the development of an early set of national nursing priorities with nurse investigators in the scientific community (Bloch, 1990). With the increased funding of nursing research since the establishment of NINR in 1986, any new priorities and themes have been advanced in the past 17 years. The priorities and themes have facilitated the focusing of scientific endeavours in nursing and the development of multiple research programmes in concentrated areas of study. This has resulted in areas of substantiated research such as the strategies for preventing premature infancy and family care-giving for elderly people. Other investigator-initiated areas of study provide the richness from which new areas of research evolve.

What are the future knowledge priorities in the USA that can be expected to influence doctoral programmes? The NINR (2003) provides one source of leadership in defining future priorities with the nursing research themes (www.nih.gov/ninr/news-info/pubs/factsht.htm, Hébert, 2003). These themes were identified through dialogue with panels of nurse researchers from the discipline's scientific community. For the next several years, five nursing research themes have been provided;

- Changing lifestyle behaviours for better health
- Managing the effects of chronic illness to improve quality of life
- Identifying effective strategies to reduce health disparities
- Harnessing advanced technologies to serve human needs
- Enhancing the end-of-life experience for patients and their families (Grady, 2003, 2000)

These research themes are reinforced in terms of importance since they reflect the social, economic, and demographic factors, and new healthcare trends discussed earlier. These priorities differ considerably from those identified for less developed countries: health of women, infant and childhood diseases and mortality concerns; assessment and management of infectious diseases; and nutrition and public health.

Canadian nurse researchers also have a strong orientation towards clinical nursing research. Jeans (1992), Dawson (1998) and CAUSN (1999) cite several areas of clinical research: assessment of the client's condition in terms of the health and illness continuum, health promotion, rehabilitative care and its effectiveness as well as long-term care. Several Canadian nurse investigators are leading scholars in the areas of human resources, work environment of nurses and the impact on patient outcomes (O'Brien-Pallas et al, 2002; Tourangeau et al, 2002).

Three major problems for nursing research in Canada are developmental in nature: insufficient numbers of well-qualified nurse investigators to conduct research, insufficient time for them to exercise their expertise, and insufficient funds and support services for researchers (CAUSN, 1999). Given these concerns, the 2002 White Paper by ACEN, AACAHO, and CASN outlines four priorities for nursing research:

- identify gaps and strategies to minimize barriers to the conduct of nursing research
- increase designated university and hospital funding for nursing research
- achieve provincial and national support to fund nursing research
- increase designated federal government funding to support nursing research.

While these four priorities focus on funding nursing research, the CASN Research Mandate (CASN/ACESI, 2003) also strongly addresses research training in several of its objectives:

- educate nurse scholars/researchers
- develop federal and international exchanges for nursing research training
- obtain increased funding for graduate education in nursing science
- provide incentives for development of 'fast-track' research-intensive graduate nursing programmes.

In summary, the nursing research priorities for Canada and the USA show consistently evolving depth and refinement in the science for nursing practice. In both countries there is continual pressure to develop the resources required for both research and research training.

Professional factors influencing knowledge development

Several professional factors have strengthened the development of knowledge to guide nursing practice in the USA and Canada. These include building strong multidisciplinary networks for developing knowledge and developing a tradition for postdoctoral study with senior nurse and multidisciplinary investigators. One factor has limited knowledge development in the discipline; this has to do with the late career stage of doctoral students and graduates, and the building of research programmes. A related factor, particularly for the near future is the anticipated shortage of nursing faculty for academic positions and roles.

Knowledge development in nursing has incorporated a strong multidisciplinary component from its early roots. The richness of the orientation of multiple disciplines, integrated and creatively used within the nursing perspective has strengthened the knowledge that can be used to guide nursing practice. In addition to enriching the knowledge base for nursing practice, interaction with other disciplines brings a new and creative scientific perspective to other non-nurse colleagues. For doctoral programmes, the strong multidisciplinary network has opened many opportunities for students and postdoctoral fellows to study with individuals of numerous fields. They are both influenced and influential in this learning process.

The development of a tradition for postdoctoral study in nursing has enhanced knowledge development in the discipline (Hinshaw and Ketefian, 1996, Hinshaw, et al, 1999). Nursing as a discipline has been late in developing this tradition. The number of postdoctoral fellows studying one to two years following their earned doctoral programmes has increased since the late 1980s in the USA and Canada. The opportunity for postdoctoral study came with the establishment of the NINR and the increase in funding for research and research training in the USA. The Canadians have been successful in competing for postdoctoral fellowships through the multiple federal agencies and foundations.

A number of nurse investigators have chosen to concentrate on building their independent research programmes with postdoctoral study. Balancing the tripartite mission of academic roles, i.e. teaching, research and service, is difficult for new faculty. Establishing the early phase of research programmes through postdoctoral work with senior nurse and multidisciplinary mentors enhances success in new academic roles and in forming strong research programmes for knowledge development.

One major problem has retarded knowledge development in the nursing discipline (Hinshaw and Ketefian, 1996; Anderson, 2000; Hinshaw, 2001). Nurses have a unique career pattern for acquiring doctoral preparation, entering quite late into doctoral programmes. The average age of the doctoral nurse student is in the late thirties and beginning assistant professors are on average 50 years of age (AACN, 2003). The demographics for Canadian nurses and scholars are similar (CNA, 1997, 2001). Since doctoral preparation provides the knowledge and skills for building research programmes and information for the discipline, this pattern of late entry into doctoral study severely limits knowledge development.

Most research and knowledge development occurs within the university and state college systems in North America. Starting a research career in the late forties or early fifties means that the scientist has approximately 15 years before retirement to build a research programme, contribute to the knowledge of the discipline, develop a reputation in healthcare based on research, and participate in health policy discussions as a leader in his or her knowledge field (Hinshaw and Ketefian, 2001). Two funded research studies, usually four years in length per study, are about all that is possible in this limited timeframe. The contribution to knowledge is thus limited.

One strategy for countering the late career issue is the establishment of rapid-progression doctoral programmes that recruit students early following their baccalaureate or Master's programmes into doctoral study. Approximately 20–25 doctoral programmes in the USA are offering a baccalaureate-to-doctoral-degree programme which allows for rapid progression through the undergraduate and graduate programmes. Because clinical experience is highly valued for the critical base provided for raising relevant nursing research questions, a number of these programmes include clinical experience in some planned form. The rapid-progression career pattern would provide doctorally prepared graduates with approximately 30–35 years of productivity as nurse investigators. Recall, the Canadian CASN objective for 'fast-tracking' faculty as well (CASN/ACESI, 2003; www.causn.org/research/casn_research_mandate.htm). The transition to this pattern will be critical in terms of the discipline's ability to develop knowledge to guide nursing practice and provide leadership from the nursing perspective for health policy at all levels.

A future limiting factor in North America will be the shortage of nursing faculty for academic positions. The shortage is expected to intensify in the next five to ten years due to the 'greying of the professoriate.' This situation is discussed in detail elsewhere in this volume. From a knowledge development perspective, the faculty shortage is likely to limit the research programmes due to a need to teach and cover more courses and advise more students.

Maintaining a strong focus and commitment of academic resources on the importance of knowledge development for the discipline and nursing research in the next decade will be critical.

Similarities and differences in knowledge development and doctoral education in the two Western regions of the globe

Knowledge development and doctoral education in the two Western, developed regions of the globe are remarkably similar in their evolution in terms of research and research training. There are also several differences based on the values and contextual factors shaping the nursing discipline's scholarship base. For the EU and the North American countries, several basic elements provide the foundation for nursing research and research training: the placement of nursing as an educational and scholarly discipline in the university and collegiate systems of the countries, the development of nursing faculty research programmes, the development of doctoral programmes, and the evolution of funding sources for nursing research and research training. For both regions, the opening of funding resources for research and research training has been a precursor to a dramatic explosion of knowledge for the practice of nursing and for doctoral and postdoctoral study.

A series of contextual factors are similar across the two regions. These factors have shaped the nursing research priorities and programmes. Nurses in many of the countries in the two regions have focused their research on critical health problems and concerns of the public that nursing, as a profession and discipline, can influence for optimal health and wellbeing. The contextual factors that are similar include:

- The Western, developed countries are all showing an 'ageing' population and thus dealing with an increasing incidence of chronic illness.
- The increasing costs of healthcare, more in the USA than in either Canada or the EU, are emphasizing health promotion and self-management of health and illness in the community settings.
- Health disparities and inequalities (by ethnicity, socioeconomic levels and gender) are evident in all the countries even though the healthcare systems are quite different. Nursing's focus on vulnerable populations makes this a clear target for nursing research.
- A pending or increasing problem with a shortage of health professionals, especially nursing, is evident in both Western regions and requires attention to both the supply or education of nurses and the retention in the healthcare work environments.

A major difference in the two Western regions is the amount of international collaboration. The structure and nature of the EU, including funding incentives and other resources, facilitates more international collaboration than between the North American countries. For Canada, and especially the USA, there are examples of international work but the structural and resource incentives are more difficult to access even though many of the research programmes focus on similar healthcare interests, such as women's health, palliative care at end-of-life and health promotion intervention studies.

The priorities for nursing research are similar across the two Western regions with several differences in terms of emphasis. For most of the countries represented, the priorities are not unlike those evident in the 2000 survey of international priorities (Hinshaw, 2000). These included health promotion across the life span, care of elderly people, shaping healthcare systems, management of symptoms secondary to illness or treatment, and quality of care outcomes balanced with cost. The survey included a number of the countries in the EU and North America.

In the past three years, a number of new priorities have evolved, responding to contextual factors and to new knowledge breakthroughs. These priorities involve:

- genetic explosion of knowledge for screening, symptom management and therapies
- multiple chronic illnesses being handled by individuals and families in the community
- palliative care and ethical issues involved with the end-of-life care
- health promotion for better lifestyles
- health disparities from multiple sources
- advanced information technology as a method for extending health and healthcare.

Several priorities are emphasized more in some countries than in others due to particular critical health needs. Studying family issues and context is a major focus in the EU and Finland, while shaping healthcare systems has been stronger in Canada due to economic and shortage of nurses' concerns. Additional research funds have targeted human resource issues in Canada and thus provide incentive for this research. Research in the USA has heavily focused on clinical research to guide nursing practice with the bulk of the funding resources in these areas of study. In the USA, an emphasis has been placed on intervention studies, while in the EU such studies are less evident but highly valued. Since intervention studies are expensive, the funding available in the USA has allowed for the increased development of these studies.

From a professional perspective, both these Western regions have similar concerns with the development of research training and the advancement of funding programmes for nursing research. Several issues and concerns about the infrastructure are evident:

- development of doctoral programmes with a special emphasis on the need for funded, senior researchers to serve as mentors and faculty
- evolution of postdoctoral study with strong nurse scientists to develop independent, funded research programmes prior to entering academic positions
- advancement of the numbers of research-prepared faculty for schools of nursing through the research training programmes
- provision of additional funding sources for nursing research and research programmes
- development of 'fast-track' doctoral programmes and other funding incentives to move nurses into doctoral programmes at a younger stage in their career.

The regions share the problem of 'greying,' older faculty who are in short supply. This has a similar impact in all the countries; a shortage of faculty compounded with a limited career in research, the ability to provide national healthcare leadership and be able to be involved in health policy decisions.

Knowledge development and doctoral education in the EU, especially Finland, and in North America, and the USA specifically, have grown dramatically in the past two decades. With the establishment of nursing doctoral and postdoctoral programmes in universities and collegiate systems, the development of strong funding sources for nursing research and research training, and the identification of priorities for nursing research, the generation of knowledge to guide nursing practice and influence the healthcare issues of the various countries has exploded. The development of nursing research programmes underlying the knowledge base is interactive with the advancement of doctoral and postdoctoral education in each country, just as the preparation of new nurse scientists feeds the development of more research and continues to advance the knowledge base. Given the identified priorities of these two developed, Western regions, the knowledge development and generation of doctoral and postdoctoral education should be even more exciting and challenging in the next decade.

References

Academy of Canadian Executive Nurses (ACEN); Association of Canadian Academic Healthcare Organizations (ACAHO); VP Research (Sub-Committee of ACAHO); Canadian Association of Schools of Nursing (CASN) (2002). *Discussion paper: Advancing a nursing research strategy in academic health science centres and teaching hospitals*, June 12, 2002; pp: 1–16.

Academy of Finland (2000). The state and quality of scientific research in Finland. *Publications of the Academy of Finland* No 7. Helsinki.

Academy of Finland (2003). PhDs in Finland: Employment, placement and demand. *Publications of the Academy of Finland* No. 5. Helsinki.

Aiken, L. H., Clarke, S. P., Sloane, D. M., et al. (2003). Hospital nurse staffing and patient mortality, nurse burnout, and job dissatisfaction. *Journal of the American Medical Association,* **289**(5), 549–551.

Alcock, D. (2002). Nurses and the Canadian Institutes of Health Research. *Canadian Journal of Nursing Research,* **34**(1), 115–117.

Algase, D. (2001). Studying fall risk factors among nursing home residents who fell. *Journal of Gerontological Nursing,* **27**(10), 26–34.

American Association of Colleges of Nursing (2003). *Fact Sheet* (AACN) http://www.aacn.nche.edu/Media/Backgrounders/facultyshortage.htm (accessed on 11/12/2003).

Anderson, C.A. (2000). Current strengths and limitations of doctoral education in nursing: Are we prepared for the future? *Journal of Professional Nursing,* **16**(4), 191–200.

Aromaa, A. (1994). Finns' health and health care seen in a European perspective. *Suomen Lääkärilehti,* **49**(15), 1623–1638.

Bloch, D. (1990). Strategies for setting and implementing the National Center for Nursing Research Priorities. *Applied Nursing Research,* 3(1), 2–6 [11 refs].

Blume, S. (1995). Problems and prospects of research training in the 1990s. In: *Research Training. Present and future.* Paris: OECD, pp: 9–30.

Browne, G., Roberts, J., Byrne, C., Gafni, A., Weir, R., and Majumdar, M. (2001). The costs and effects of addressing the needs of vulnerable populations: Results of 10 years of research. *Canadian Journal of Nursing Research,* **33**(1), 65–76.

Buerhaus, P. I. (2000). A nursing shortage with a fundamental difference. Syllabus. *American Association of Colleges of Nursing,* **26**(5), 3–4, 7.

Butler, L., Love, B., Reimer, M. et al. (2002). Nurses begin a national plan for the integration of supportive care in health research, practice, and policy. *Canadian Journal of Nursing Research,* **33**(4), 155–169.

Callahan, D. (1985). Ethics and health care: The next 20 years. *American Journal of Hospital Pharmacy,* **42**, 1053–1057.

Canadian Association of Schools of Nursing/ACESI (2003). http://www.causn.org/research/casn_research_mandate.htm (accessed on 11/12/2003).

Canadian Association of University Schools of Nursing (1999). A concept of research in the University. *Canadian Journal of Nursing Research,* **30**(4), 159–164.

Canadian Nurses Association (1997). *Doctoral and post-doctoral preparation in nursing.* CNA policy statement, approved by the Board of Directors, November. http://www.cna-nurses.ca/pages/policies/doctor_prep.html (accessed on 11/12/2003).

Canadian Nurses Association (2001). Registered nurses 2001 statistical highlights. Canadian Institute for Health Information. www.cna-nurses.ca/_frames/search frame.htm (accessed on 11.12.2003).

Dawson, P. (1998). Realizing the imperative of clinical nursing research: the experiences of a collaborative research program in long-term care. *Canadian Journal of Nursing Research,* **30**(2), 125–134.

Elomaa, L. (2003). *Research evidence implementation and its requirements in nursing education.* Finland: Annales Universitatis Turkuensis, University of Turku.

Eriksson, K. (1997). Finland. In: E. Hamrin and M. Lorensen (eds). *Perspectives on priorities in nursing science. Vårdalstiftelsens rapportserie* No 1, Stockholm, pp: 29–39.

European Academy for Nursing (2003). www.eans.org (accessed on 20.7.2003). http://www.ecn.nl/ps/index.en.html ECN policy studies (accessed on 18.7.2003).

European Commission (2000). *Report on the state of young people's health in the European Union. A Commission Services Working Paper.* Brussels: Directorate General Health and Consumer Protection.

European Commission (2003). *The health status of the European Union, Narrowing the health gap.* Luxembourg: Office for Official Publications of the European Communities.

European Commission, Public Health. http://europa.eu.int/comm/health/ (accessed on 18.8.2003.

European Observatory on Health Care Systems (2002). *Health care systems in eight countries: trends and challenges.* A. Dixon and E. Mossialos (eds). London: The London School of Economics and Political Science.

Eurostat (2003a). Statistics in focus, Population and social conditions, No 8/2003. Poverty and social exclusion in the EU after Laeken – part 1. www.europa.eu.int/comm/eurostat.

Eurostat (2003b). Statistics in focus, Population and social conditions, No 9/2003. Poverty and social exclusion in the EU after Laeken – part 2. www.europa.eu.int/comm/eurostat.

Evers, G. (2003). Developing nursing science in Europe. *Journal of Nursing Scholarship*, First Quarter, 9–13.

Frijdal, A. and Bartelse, J. (eds) (1999). *The future of postgraduate education in Europe.* Luxembourg: European Commission.

Grady, P. A. (2003). *Report of the National Institute of Nursing Research. National Research Council Project: Monitoring the Changing Needs for Biomedical and Behavioral Research Personnel.* Bethesda, MD: NINR.

Grady, P. A. (2000). http://www.nih.gov/ninr/research/themes.doc; http://www.nih.gov/ninr/research/diversity/mission.html.

Hamrin, E. (1990). Nursing research in Sweden. *International Journal of Nursing Studies,* **27**(2), 149–158.

Hamrin, E. (1997). *Models of Doctoral Education in Europe.* Paper presented at the Conference of the International Network for Doctoral Education in Nursing: Vision and Strategy for International Doctoral Education, June, 1997, Vancouver, Canada. www. umich.edu/~inden.

Hamrin, E. and Lorensen, M. (eds) (1997). Perspectives on priorities in nursing science. *Vårdalstiftelsens rapportserie* No 1/1197, Solna: Williamssons.

Hébert, R. (2003). NINR sleep research means wake-up call for policy. *American Psychological Society Observer,* **16** (7), 19–29.

Hicks, P. (1996). The impact of aging on public policy. *The OECD Observer*, No 203, December 1996/January 1997, 19–21.

Hinshaw, A. S. (1999). Evolving nursing research traditions: influencing factors. In: A. S. Hinshaw, S. L. Feetham, and J. L. Shaver (Eds). *Handbook of clinical nursing research.* Thousand Oaks, CA: Sage Publications, 19–31.

Hinshaw, A. S. (2000). Nursing knowledge for the 21st century: Opportunities and challenges. *Journal of Nursing Scholarship,* **32**(2), 117–123.

Hinshaw, A. S. (2001). A continuing challenge: the shortage of educationally prepared nursing faculty. *Online Journal of Issues of Nursing,* **6**(1), 14 [24 ref].

Hinshaw, A. S. and Ketefian, S. (1996). A missing research tradition. *Journal of Professional Nursing*, **12** (4), 196 [editorial].

Hinshaw, A.S. and Ketefian, S. (2001). Nurse scientist preparation: Fast track for academic nursing. In: *Envisioning doctoral education for the future*. Washington, DC: American Association of Colleges of Nursing, pp. 63–75.

Hinshaw, A. S., Feetham, S. L., and Shaver, J. L. (ed) (1999). *Handbook of clinical nursing research*. Thousand Oaks, CA: Sage Publications.

Hoitotiede-lehti (1999). Special issue describing research programmes in five Finnish universities. *Finnish Journal of Nursing Science,* **11**(6), 311–364 [In Finnish; English abstract].

Institute of Medicine (1997a). *Approaching death; Improving care at the end of life.* Washington, DC: National Academy Press.

Institute of Medicine (1997b). *Managing managed care: Quality improvement in behavioral health.* Washington, DC: National Academy Press.

Institute of Medicine (2003a). *Unequal treatment: Confronting racial and ethnic disparities in health care.* Washington, DC: The National Academy Press.

Institute of Medicine (2003b). *A Shared Destiny.* Washington, DC: The National Academy Press.

Institute of Medicine (2003c). *Keeping patients safe: Transforming the work environment of nurses.* Washington DC: National Academy Press.

Institute of Medicine (2002). *Health insurance is a family matter.* Washington, DC: National Academy Press.

International Council of Nurses (2003). http://icn.ch/index.html (accessed 11/12/2003).

Jackson, S. A., Shiferaw, B., Anderson, R. T., Heuser, M. D., Hutchinson, K. M., and Mittelmark, M. B. (2002). Racial differences in service utilization: the Forsyth County Aging Study. *Journal of Health Care for the Poor and Underserved,* **13**(3), 320–33.

Jeans, M. E. (1992). Clinical significance of research: A growing concern. *Canadian Journal of Nursing Research,* **24**(1), 1–2.

Jonsdottir, H. (2001). Chronic illness. *Scandinavian Journal of Caring Sciences,* **15**(1), 1–2 [Editorial].

Ketefian, S. and Redman, R.W. (1997). Nursing science in the global community. *Image: Journal of Nursing Scholarship,* **29**(1), 11–15.

Lauri, S. (1990). The history of nursing research in Finland. *International Journal of Nursing Studies,* **27**(2), 169–173.

Leino-Kilpi, H. and Suominen, T. (1998). Nursing research in Finland from 1958 to 1995. *Image, Journal of Nursing Scholarship,* **30**(4), 363–367.

Leino-Kilpi, H. and Uski, A. (2001). Nursing education in Finland. In: C. Begley and J. Roode (eds). *Nurse educators/leaders from European Union countries in international partnership, Part 2.* The Netherlands: International Society for University Nurses.

Leino-Kilpi, H., Välimäki, M., Arndt, M. et al. (2000). Patients' autonomy, privacy and informed consent. *Biomedical and Health Research.* Amsterdam: IOS Press.

Lerheim. K. (1990). Nursing research developments in Norway. *International Journal of Nursing Studies,* **27**(2), 139–148.

Lorensen, M. (1990). Research resource development in Denmark. *International Journal of Nursing Studies,* **27** (2), 159–168.

McClure, M. and Hinshaw, A. S. (2002). *Magnet hospitals revisited: Attraction and retention of professional nurses.* Washington, DC: American Nurses Publishing (American Academy of Nursing).

McKenna, H. and Cutcliffe, J. (2001). Nursing doctoral education in the United Kingdom and Ireland. *Online Journal of Issues in Nursing*, **5**(2), www.nursing world.org (accessed on 11/12/2003).

Merritt, D. H. (1986). The National Center for Nursing Research. *Image: Journal of Nursing Scholarship*, **18**(3), 84–85.

Ministry of Education (2000). *The graduate school system in Finland. Survey of functioning, results and efficiency by 2000*. Helsinki, Finland: Ministry of Education.

National Institute of Nursing Research (2003). Fact Sheet. http://www.nih.gov/ninr/news-info/pubs/factsht.htm (accessed on 11/12/2003).

Noble, K. (1994). *Changing doctoral degrees: An international perspective*. Bristol: Open University Press.

Nyquist, J. (2002). The PhD: A tapestry of change for the 21st century. *Change*, **34**(6), 12–20.

O'Brien-Pallas, L. L., Irvine, D. D., Murray, M. et al. (2002). Evaluation of a client care delivery model, Part 2: Variability in client outcomes in community home nursing. *Nursing Economic$*, **20**(1), 13–21, 36.

Organisation for Economic Co-operation and Development (1991). *Postgraduate education today: Changing structures for a changing Europe*. Paris: OECD.

OECD (1995). *Research training. Present and future*. Paris: OECD.

OECD (2001). *Aging and income: Financial resources and retirement in 9 OECD countries*. Paris: OECD.

OECD (2002). *Measuring the information economy*. Paris: OECD.

OECD (2003). *Health Data*. www.oecd.fr (accessed on 15.8.2003).

Perälä, M.L. (ed.) (1998). *The direction of nursing: A strategy for quality and effectiveness, project group of nursing*. Stakes, Helsinki: Ministry of Social Affairs and Health.

Rahm-Hallberg, I. (2003). *Quality development in the nurses' doctoral education from a Swedish perspective*. www.umich.edu/inden/papers/models.html.

Segersten, K. (1993). Articles published in *Scandinavian Journal of Caring Sciences* between 1987 and 1991. *Scandinavian Journal of Caring Sciences* **4**, 195–199.

Sinkkonen, S. (1988). University education in caring sciences in Finland. *Scandinavian Journal of Caring Sciences*, **2**(2), 51–55.

Sternberg, S. (2001). Race, locale raise men's heart risk: Study reflects societal 'defects.' *USA Today*, June 21, pp: A01.

Stewart, M. (1997). Centres for health promotion research in Canada. *Canadian Journal of Nursing Research*, **29**(3), 111.

Stewart, M. J., Kushner, K. E. and Spitzer D. L. (2001). Research priorities in gender and health. *Canadian Journal of Nursing Research*, **33**(3), 5–15.

Strack, G. (2003). Towards a European knowledge-based society: the contributions of men and women. *Statistics in focus, science and technology*, Theme 9, 5/2003. www.europa.eu.int/comm/eurostat.

Suominen, T. and Leino-Kilpi, H. (1998). Review of Finnish nursing research from 1958 to 1995. *Scandinavian Journal of Caring Sciences*, **12**, 57–62.

Tierney, A. J. (1997). Organization report. The development of nursing research in Europe. *European Nurse* **2**(2), 73–84.

Tomlinson, P. and Hall, E. (2003). Expanding knowledge in family health care. *Scandinavian Journal of Caring Sciences*, **17**(2), 93–95. [Guest editorial].

Tourangeau, A. E., Giovannetti, P., Tu, J.V. and Wood, M. (2002). Nursing-related determinants of 30-day mortality for hospitalized patients. *Canadian Journal of Nursing Research*, **33**(4), 71–88.

Van Maanen, H. (1998). *Review of 20 years development of nursing research in the countries of the European Region 1997*. Germany: University of Bremen.

Waidmann, T. A. and Rajan, S. (2000). Race and ethnic disparities in health care access utilization: An examination of state variation. *Medical Care Research and Review*, **57**, Suppl 1, 55–84.

Villarruel, A. M. (2001). *MESA center for health disparities grant*. Bethesda, MD: NIH/NINR.

Workgroup of European Nurse Researchers (1997). *Nursing research report and recommendations*. Initial review, submitted to Standing Committee of Nurses of the European Union.

WENR (2003). *A position paper: Nursing research in Europe*. www.wenr.org (accessed on 24.7.2003).

World Health Organization (1999). *Health21 – health for all in the 21st century. European Health for All*, Series No 6, Copenhagen: WHO Regional Office for Europe. www.who.dk.

WHO (2002). *Building the evidence base of the nursing and midwifery contribution to health*. WHO Regional Office for Europe, Copenhagen. www.who.dk.

Working Group for the Study of Ethical Issues in International Nursing Research (Chair Douglas P. Olsen) (2003). Ethical considerations in international nursing research: A report from the International Center for Nursing Ethics. *Nursing Ethics*, **10** (2), 122–137.

www.europa.eu.int/comm/eurostat (accessed on 17.8.2003. http://europa.eu.int/comm/eurostat/Public/datashop/printcatalogue/EN?catalogue=Eurostat.

www.europa.eu.int/comm/health (accessed on 30.7.2003).

www.finlex.fi (accessed on 15.7.2003).

www.ocenf.org (accessed on 18.8.2003). The European Forum of National Nursing and Midwifery Associations and WHO, November, 2003.

www.oecd.fr (accessed on 15.8 and on 18.8.2003). http://www.oecd.fr/home/ Organization for Economic Co-operation and Development.

www.wenr.org (accessed on 18.8.2003). http://www.wes.org/ewenr/03sept/index.asp. World Education News and Reviews.

www.who.int (accessed on 19.8.2003). http://www.who.int/en/. World Health Organization.

Chapter 3

Doctoral education for transformational leadership in a global context

Gwen D Sherwood and Dawn Freshwater

The pace of change in the world is unprecedented, calling for nurse leaders who are responsive to new workplace environments, which require new strategies that question prevailing assumptions. Doctoral education in nursing must be reframed to prepare leaders with new skills to transform the organizational culture in which care delivery takes place. Leaders must be able to analyse trends in the healthcare market, manage growing diversity, and incorporate emerging evidence about the workplace. Doctoral education is charged with preparing leaders who can think out of the box and stimulate creative problem solving in others, invigorating nurses to claim a voice in crafting a vision of healthcare delivery that recognizes the essentialness of nursing.

What are the essential elements of doctoral education that promote and enable transformation, that changing of the worldview which offers the ability to lead in a dynamic way? Leadership that can move people as well as organizations to transformation is a key strategy for advancing nursing in a global context. It becomes an essential component of nursing doctoral curricula in the rapidly developing global healthcare environment. Traditional leadership models are giving way to dynamic approaches that focus on personal development as the core ingredient of the leadership journey. This new vision for professional development based on critical reflection allows one to understand individual differences, the context in which nursing practice takes place, and the organizational culture that influences transformational changes. Transformational leadership can produce quality outcomes for patients as well as for nurses.

Imperative for change amid global challenges

Nursing has been challenged by the label of silent profession. Historical developments related to views of nursing as a calling, symbol of the angel of mercy, socialization associated with being a predominantly female profession, environments entrenched in steep hierarchy, and other societal factors have contributed to the lack of voice attributed to nurses in the decision-making arena that drives the healthcare market. The convergence of many factors offers new opportunities that perhaps are best met with preparation of new leadership skills in doctoral education. A view of nursing that recognizes each nurse as a leader requires new approaches to leadership development and changes in doctoral curricula.

Evolution in healthcare

This is a dynamic era in which healthcare systems are evolving worldwide, opening an opportunity for increased attention to nursing brought by the challenges of a global shortage of nurses to meet patient care needs. Analysis of the context of healthcare delivery confirms the leadership potential for nurses. Nurses are the discipline present with patients around the clock, and the discipline charged with coordinating care among all the disciplines. Globalization has brought the world community together, as technology expands and information exchange happens instantly. Nurses communicate around the globe on a daily basis, sharing information, coaching and mentoring, and expanding research opportunities for evidence-based practice. In fact, education is no longer delivered only in synchronous modes, but instead, is frequently delivered on demand using various delivery modes.

The exponential growth of medical and technological advances has changed the way healthcare operates with an overwhelming knowledge expansion. It is no longer what one knows, but how well and how quickly one can retrieve the required information. Nursing curricula have to move from content-driven to new models based on integration and synthesis within a critical thinking modality. The twenty-first century learner is action-oriented, calling for new delivery methods with fewer boundaries, given the proliferation of technology-driven programmes. These shifts have the nursing faculty in stages of change, while addressing the dual challenges of how classes are to be delivered, and revamping what is delivered, the changing curriculum itself.

Changing the work environment is a new wave recruitment and retention strategy helping propel nursing beyond the blue-collar syndrome in which nurses were compensated based on an hourly wage. Similar to other professions that are moving beyond the industrial age, nursing is primed for new leadership strategies that foster transformational changes in education, service delivery, work environments, recruitment and retention, and performance-based compensation. The new generation of nurses, most born after the technology revolution began in the 1970s, have always lived in a world of technology, and so respond to leadership approaches that recognize their individuality, and motivate and inspire (Zemke et al, 2000). This generation can, with exposure to transformational leaders, help move nursing from silence to voice. What, then, is the role of doctoral education in making the changes that are needed?

Moving towards transformational change

It is argued in many parts of the world that leadership within nursing is receiving unprecedented focus and development (Graham, 2003). Traditional leadership methods have focused on managing people, how-to strategies and management theories. Emerging leadership approaches have evolved from self-development as a central component of the leadership journey. By creating a new vision for professional growth, one can begin to understand the significance of the influence of individual differences, context, organization and culture (Cranton, 1996). Even as Porter-O'Grady and Malloch (2003) warn of the end of the current era of nursing education and practice as known by current practitioners and educators, changes are evident. New skills are imperative to survive in the rapidly developing interdisciplinary arena. The nature of nursing and nursing work is changing around the globe. New leadership models must seize the moment to lead nursing into the evolving healthcare arena, challenging the nurse educators who prepare the new generations of leaders.

Traditional leadership models

Traditional approaches to leadership in nursing have been centred around transactional models. Such models are being challenged, with Thyer (2003) contesting that a transactional style of leadership, as opposed to a transformational approach, potentially contributes to the high attrition rates within the profession. In her recent study, she provides specific examples of the impact of transactional leadership and contrasts them with what might result if a transformational leadership model was embraced.

Principles of transformation

Leadership approaches for twenty-first century nursing can be considered to fit the process of individual transformation described in three stages by Cranton (1996): self-directed learning, critical reflection and transformative learning. Self-directed learning sets the foundation for transformation as the learner takes responsibility and accountability for the process rather in contrast with the teacher-controlled, content-driven approach used by traditional lecture-only educators. In this dialogical process, the teacher and learner share mutual work together. The learner moves forward through critical reflection to learn from experience by recalling, reflecting, analysing, theorizing, and recontextualizing to arrive at new conclusions and behaviours through understanding. The final stage is the application through transformative learning. Here, through critical self-reflection in the inward journey of self-discovery, the learner articulates assumptions and questions those assumptions to move into meaningful perspectives.

Applied to leadership, the transformational process takes the learner into the inward journey of self-awareness. The journey of leadership is defined as a journey of self-development; no leader is stronger than his or her inner core of the person, honed through character, commitment, connectedness, compassion and confidence (Kowalski and Yoder-Wise, 2003). Leaders have primarily been taught to manage people; twenty-first century leadership demands that leaders motivate and manage movements to achieve lasting change. Leading the movement of change demands a critically reflective practitioner, and an individual who is willing to engage in a constant critical dialogue with their practice. In this way transformational leadership becomes associated with healthcare improvement, what Graham (2003) describes as the cornerstone of clinical leadership.

Transformational leadership helps capture the elusive quality of leadership, the inner strength and character cultivated through critical reflection of experiences, particularly those based on difficult circumstances that test one's mettle. In managing movements, leaders manage dynamism, requiring that they be dynamic themselves (Porter-O'Grady and Malloch, 2003). Trofino (1995) concurs with this view, stating that healthcare situations require leaders who develop individuals committed to action, convert and empower followers, and transform leaders into change agents.

Key concepts in doctoral curricula strengthen the ability to apply principles of change as the foundation for leadership development that strives to unleash entrenched assumptions and management patterns. Transformational leaders must themselves understand the basics of change as well as lead others into the change process, thus transforming circumstances. The first stage in the process is recognizing the need for change leading to different ways of thinking and performing. Unfreezing old behaviours requires unbundling assumptions, departing from tradition and questioning why something is the way it is. Change is itself a continuum and moves from recognition of the need to identifying possibilities and designing new approaches, methods, or ways to think or act. Transformation results as new patterns are embraced and become part of the routine.

Reinforcing and maintaining change is a difficult stage as people have a tendency to revert back to former, entrenched behaviours. It is important in the recognizing stage for those involved to have the time and direction for critical reflection to internalize the need for change, e.g. the necessity of understanding the improved outcome that will result from the change. Real change and growth is an on-going process of examining and questioning assumptions, values and perspectives. A pervasive attitude of continual advancement thus revitalizes the workplace so that it is a dynamic environment attracting the best minds. The ability of the leader to manage such movement is an embedded skill of the transformational leader (Porter-O'Grady and Malloch, 2003).

The challenge for doctoral education is designing learning activities to apply the processes critical to transformational leadership as well as determining essential content strands. The preceding sections presented the challenges to leadership in the current environment and described the process for preparing leaders. The following discussion examines a framework for preparing transformational leaders.

An emerging leadership paradigm in doctoral education

Doctoral educators are themselves challenged by the rapid change in healthcare delivery and application of organizational development gleaned from the business world. An examination of organizational culture sets the stage for emerging leadership for the twenty-first century offering a framework for doctoral curricula. While most examples relate to the practice arena, the same principles apply to the academic settings for nursing education where leadership is an essential curriculum topic.

Organizational culture

One goal of doctoral education is to create a shift in the worldview of the doctoral student so that they move beyond the individual to consider the organizational context. Transformational leadership requires a systems thinking approach able to deconstruct the organizational context in which care delivery occurs. Analysis of context begins with understanding the organization's culture – regardless of its location in the world, every organization has a culture which derives from the way the stated philosophy is actualized in the workplace. It is influenced by how well the stated philosophy is matched by everyday reality at the point of service (Bolman and Deal, 1997). It is first modelled by institutional leaders; a healthy organization maintains the same standards for top leadership and for those delivering services at all levels of the organization. This point poses a challenge for academia: finding sufficient faculty prepared to teach from an updated curriculum, made more poignant by the critical faculty shortage of the early twenty-first century. Most current faculty are themselves new learners of the emerging transformational leadership paradigm, having been schooled in more traditional approaches.

The new generation nurse leaders must be able to move outside traditional hierarchical models of leadership to balance economic needs of the organization with employee motivation, satisfaction and morale, and quality outcomes. Values management recognizes that expert staff or experienced faculty are an essential yet scarce resource such that each worker becomes important in providing adequate services. The challenges of developing responsive leaders to manage the shifting healthcare environment demand re-examination of the leadership paradigm and the underlying assumptions.

Curricula threads examining organizational context lead to analysis of various factors influencing the workplace. There is increasing global awareness of key factors in workplace satisfaction. The first factor is how involved and engaged nurses are in the work they do. Being present and engaged in one's task can offer deep satisfaction. Secondly, administrators must be willing to change from supervision to facilitation in which workers are enabled and motivated to accomplish work effectively, that is, they own their responsibilities and are accountable for the outcomes (Bolman and Deal, 1997). The reality is that the prevailing emphasis on efficiency and economics encourages micromanagement for output such that employees often feeling depersonalized is a commodity in the budget. Organizational culture affects satisfaction, which affects retention, and ultimately influences recruitment. Workplace culture is significant, yet few healthcare providers understand how to shape the environment for their workers' engagement, health and satisfaction.

A critical role of the leader is knowing how to create and manage the work environment as well as deconstruct the culture when needed (Jones and Redman, 2000). Culture is built from shared values and group behaviour norms. Values influence decisions that lead to group behaviour norms, common ways of acting among group members that persist as they are reinforced by group members; the connection between behaviour and its consequences contributes to the culture. When personal values fail to match those of the organization, there is dissonance and dissatisfaction. Herein lies a strategic component for doctoral education in preparing the new generations of leaders. Changing the culture means changing behaviours to match philosophy, mission and values to everyday work, difficult under any circumstances.

Leaders create strength in adaptive organizations by constantly reinforcing mission, goals, and strategies so that all workers know what is important and how things are done (Jones and Redman, 2000). Those working closest to the patient or the point of service are the ones who are the heart of an organization. Leaders must remember that the needs of workers are as important as the needs of customers; both serve the needs of the organization.

Leaders must be prepared to face barriers to a healthy culture: centralized leadership, poor communication, powerlessness, alienation, reliance on policy and procedure, and workplace stress (Grindel et al, 1996). Evidence indicates that a healthy workplace culture is linked with autonomy, communication with direct managers and peers, and recognition or feedback for good work, and contributes to physical and mental wellbeing of the patients and staff, thus playing a role in healthy outcomes for both.

Changes in healthcare leadership

If it is to change, the healthcare workplace needs a new leadership paradigm that can ensure meaningful work and reduce fragmentation and shortages (American Hospital Association, 2002). Increasing patient acuity coincided with personnel shortages, thus overloading the workforce contributing to the disillusionment that is part of the poor image of nursing as a profession (Sherwood, 2003). Traditional management-based leadership has been challenged to move the organization to focus on mission and values-based healthcare. The healthcare market is driven by economics and outcomes, shifting the emphasis of nursing to decreasing length of hospital stay and measuring quality benchmarks against industry leaders to determine outcomes of care. Nursing shortages, medical errors, poor image, a greying work force, declining numbers, and poor compensation contribute to poor morale in many countries around the globe, not solved by past leadership strategies. Continuing the same strategies will not change the results (Porter-O'Grady and Malloch, 2003).

Nurse leaders with knowledge of how organizations work have the opportunity to reshape the structure and influence the culture (Laschinger et al, 2000). 'Each nurse a leader' means each nurse uses his or her sphere of influence, wherever they are in their work setting, to move the profession forward, to offer administrative leadership, to lead teams of workers in delivery of care, to mentor and guide students, to shape policy, or to advocate for patients. Claiming voice means learning techniques for productive interdisciplinary communication, speaking up for what is right and just, guiding patients through the healthcare maze, and influencing policy formation and curriculum decisions. Wherever the nurse works, there is opportunity for leadership, often unclaimed. Changing the way we prepare leaders so that we build from the inner core of the person can produce a new generation of leaders for the profession.

Sherwood et al (2002) called for a relational model of leadership to build teamwork, requiring a new kind of provider skilled in the art and science of nursing. Leadership as an art and a science melds accountability based on responsibility, connecting through relationships, reverence that respects each individual, and exchange of knowledge for care delivery. Relational leadership is built through development of emotional competencies including self-awareness, self-regulation, self-motivation and empathy. Relationship skills help to collaborate and communicate with others while influencing and managing conflict, and building consensus and support. The four cornerstones of partnerships described by Parker and Gadbois (2000) sum up the developmental process of a relational model of leadership: seeing oneself differently through inner self-discovery; seeing others differently as a community connected through dialogue and communication; seeing power differently with a balance of influence and integrated, value-based decision making; and seeing the whole differently with a shift from mechanistic to organic with revamped values, mission and vision.

In summary, leadership that guides an organization through turbulent times must be able to break out of the box to see a new version of the present reality, thus viewing the workplace and its workers with a new lens. Transformational leaders create the possibility of building a culture that promotes the autonomy, communication and recognition that foster a satisfied workforce. Doctoral educators have the task of developing curricular models based on the emerging leader paradigm and moving from the traditional transactional model towards one of transformation.

Doctoral education developing leadership as a journey of the self

In the silent voice mode, nurses have often assumed that 'someone else can do it', yet each nurse has a responsibility to be a leader in shaping the environment. Adaptation of doctoral curricula explores how any change process begins with the individual and expands in the circle of influence. Transformational leadership, leaders who create lasting change, begins then as a journey of the self (Bolman and Deal, 2001). Leadership derives from giving one's self and spirit, propelling a reciprocal process as others give of themselves in return. Each person and their individual development into self-awareness are the focus of effective leadership. Emotionally intelligent leaders develop self-awareness, searching for the true self (Vitello-Cicciu, 2002). The workplace is transformed only as the leader transforms his or her own self, nurturing spirit in the organization by inspiring each worker to begin their own journey.

Emotional intelligence and transformational leadership

Emerging doctoral curricula weave difficult concepts of a new leadership paradigm based on self-awareness. The concept of emotional intelligence has grown in popularity over the past two decades, generating interest both at a social and a professional level. Concurrent developments in nursing relate to the recognition of the impact of self-awareness and reflexive practice on the quality of the patient experience and the drive towards evidence-based, patient-centred models of care. Many curricula now make reference in some way to the notion of an emotionally intelligent practitioner, one for whom theory, practice and research are inextricably bound up with tacit and experiential knowledge.

Every nursing intervention is affected by the master aptitude of emotional intelligence. While the rational mind may adequately attend to the necessary technical aspects of nursing procedures, it is not the place of the rational mind to intuitively sense the needs and emotions of the person at the receiving end of care (Freshwater and Stickley, in press). Bellack (1999) argues for nurses to develop emotional competence if they are to be successful in their working environment. Citing that nurse education fails in the important domain of the emotions, Bellack (1999) calls for nurse educators to examine the role of emotional learning and competencies within the curricula. The role of nursing education in supporting this development is as yet unclear, although it would appear from the literature that there are some initiatives that specifically aim to explore the link between emotional intelligence and the nursing curricula (Bellack, 1999; Cadman and Brewer, 2001; Evans and Allen, 2002). What is clear is that transformational leaders and professional practitioners require a degree of emotional intelligence to inspire and facilitate movement. Planners of doctoral curricula are urged to be mindful of the power of emotional intelligence when developing innovative and creative ways of delivering teaching and learning at this level.

Balance in organizations

New concepts for doctoral curricula surround individual development within an organizational context. Organizations seek balance even in the midst of turbulent times. An innovative approach from Bolman and Deal (2001) describes four dualities – caring and power, and authorship and significance – that offer balance in an organization. As individuals in the organization master any of the dualities, opposites that make each other possible, organizations gain harmony and balance. For instance, the dualities of caring and power are described using the Chinese concept of yin and yang. Yin is associated with the more feminine principle for caring and compassion, while the more male principle, yang, describes power with autonomy and influence. Authorship is connected with individual accomplishment and craftsmanship, while significance surfaces through meaning, unity and pride. These four dualities comprise the spirit of an organization and ignite the unique synergy of a leadership paradigm that can transform the workplace (Bolman and Deal, 2001).

Dualities in leadership development

The dualities of caring and power can be further applied to nursing leadership, describing essential skills in a doctoral curriculum. Caring is a core value and unifying force in nursing (Sherwood, 1997). Self-awareness offers inner security for the openness to know the other through listening, understanding and acceptance with presence for one another and caring enough to see the real person. Trust inspires giving of self. Workers who feel cared about give caring back to both coworkers and patients in a reciprocal pattern (Bolman and Deal, 2001).

Power is perhaps the most difficult concept to convey. Power is not about control but the ability to influence others. Power is particularly important in an education context. Faculty must beware of the implicit power that governs much of the student–teacher relationship. This view of power is consistent with dialogical modes of teaching, a mutual process of discovery engaging both teacher and learner, not one in which the teacher exerts undue influence from the threat of evaluation of the student.

Productive empowerment creates a culture of inclusion and participation in the processes affecting staff or faculty and derives from trust, listening, asking questions and knowing what is happening. Together the dualities of authorship and significance give workers a connection to their work, contributing to their experience of meaning and purpose. By encouraging creativity and craftsmanship, staff put signature on their work. Authorship is owning one's work. The connection to one's work is essential to satisfaction and renewal. Leaders have the responsibility to create conditions for authorship that help people feel they have the power to complete their work and thus feel personally accountable. Autonomy in the workplace offers satisfaction from meaningful accomplishments. Leaders who let go of control, lead, rather than manage, knowing staff will invest in the outcome through ownership and accountability. Leaders need the ability to coach, mentor, and offer direction to help others learn a framework for making decisions, providing space yet setting boundaries.

What are strategies to stimulate worker engagement? Workers vested in outcomes gain significance from their work. Leaders who impart significance help employees feel unity, pride and meaning. Significance is at the core of interpersonal relationships and interdependence. Pride arises from the satisfaction of contributing to something of lasting value, of making a difference in the world and from creating outcomes together so that workers are eager to come to work. Delivery systems, economic pressures and staff shortages diminish significance, leaving healthcare workers feeling dissatisfied even though their work is inherently meaningful. It is the task of the leader to foster significance by ensuring adequate resources, growth opportunities, and involvement at all levels.

Reflective learning: an ingredient in doctoral curricula

What would a doctoral programme look like that fosters transformational leadership? Learners must become involved in the process, not just absorb content. Transformation is changing of worldview, taking on new ways of collecting information, synthesizing and recontextualizing to find new meanings of one's work. It is not taking on knowledge as information only, but rather it is taking accountability for one's learning so that the search becomes one of finding what one needs to know to solve difficult situations, analyse organizational context, or advance nursing knowledge.

Discovering meaning

Meaning derives from reflection on creative work in which one must confront fears, break old patterns and seek self-discovery. It requires reflective evaluation of oneself, looking at one's potential, preferred direction, repressed hopes and fantasies of the future. Emotionally intelligent workers strive towards self-transcendence by getting outside the self to help others with commitment to a cause greater than the self (Vitello-Cicciu, 2002).

Creating context

The role of the nurse leader in the healthcare arena is to create context for nursing practice. Leaders share in achieving mission at all levels of the organization, whether in a practice setting or in academia. Purpose-driven workers encounter new situations with new potentials by honouring values and mission. Healthcare constantly balances competing values and demands while honouring mission and ensuring survival, making tough decisions amid tight resources.

Reflection on action

Other skills required of transformational leaders include reflective practice to enable other practitioners to identify the contradictions between desired practice and actual practice. If doctoral programmes are to develop transformational leaders there must be fundamental changes in the thinking, philosophy and delivery of the curriculum or the educational model to include the processes of both reflective practice and critical reflection.

Although most postgraduate courses necessitate a degree of reflective practice, not all of them foster the more indepth and rigorous processes of critical reflection and reflexivity (Freshwater and Rolfe, 2001; Rolfe et al, 2001). Freshwater (2003) defines reflective practice as 'thinking about your practice,' with critical reflection requiring that the individual 'thinks about how they are thinking about their practice.' That is to say that the practitioner is reflecting upon his or her reflections, while being mindful of the influences of the dominant discourses within which they are operating.

Recognizing, understanding and challenging the ways in which the historical, social, political and ethical context of professional practice is informed by and informs clinical decision-making processes facilitates the development of a leader who models a practitioner/researcher-based approach to improving and developing practice (Freshwater and Rolfe, 2001). Reflection is a problem-solving, intuitive process using interaction and a developmental process leading to transformation to see expectations of self and those in their influence and the larger worldview.

Willing engagement

Fostering willing engagement is a skill of transformational leaders; they see that quality in others and nurture it. To impart this in a doctoral programme, faculty must first model willing engagement in the teaching–learning process. Faculty who are engaged in the scholarly pursuit of nursing become mentors and coaches for willing engagement, inspiring students to likewise invest in their own learning and translate the attitude of willing engagement into their practice.

Transformative leadership connects the leader with those they influence, the knowledge with the leader in a meaningful and purposeful context to move beyond managing things and people to interpretative actions that shift and promote lasting change. This goes beyond techniques and how-to, delving to deeper reflection on the meaning and vision of the whole of their work. Transformative leaders inherently connect with the meaning and purpose of their work.

Finding the internal compass

In order to connect with the meaning and purpose of their work, doctoral candidates initially need to focus on the self through reflective practice.

Re-establishing and re-evaluating their own personal internalized beliefs, values and norms to define and describe their own philosophical stance towards nursing practice and indeed, practise improvement and leadership. Leadership then begins with the self, using reflective practice to locate the internal compass by which the practitioner is guided (Freshwater, 2003). That inner core of being, called the internal compass, guides and directs actions and practices, fuelled from one's values and spirituality of meaning. When it becomes the central voice of a person, it is the inspiration for greatness and 'doing the right thing'.

Although reflection on the self is an important feature of doctoral level education, it must always be done within the context of other. This is to say that reflection, when utilized with critical intent, is a dialogic process and in this sense doctoral education enables the individual to move between the universal and the particular (Freshwater, 2002). The role of the doctoral educator shifts from one that supplies knowledge in a didactic manner, in which the learner is passively part of the educational process. The doctoral educator moves into a participatory style of teaching, coaching, and mentoring, in which the learner becomes a partner, building on previous knowledge and skills. As teacher and learner work together, the process becomes dialogical as the student drives his or her own learning. The path will vary for each student as they move through the discovery and understanding of their own learning needs, building from their foundation uncovered from reflection. This journey of the self becomes a critical aspect of the transformation journey in doctoral education as the learner dwells on their own way of practice, being, and doing in a dynamic continuum of growth and development.

Where reflective learning can herald a movement towards professional artistry, and the ability to respond spontaneously to complex and often contradictory sets of circumstances, change and transformation are the main intent of critical reflection and reflexivity. These skills are linked to mindfulness: presence/attentiveness to the moment and the concept of willingness/engagement, and to creating a healthy, nurturing but challenging working environment.

Summary and conclusions

What goes into doctoral education that promotes or enables transformation, the changing of worldview and ability to lead in a dynamic way? Changes in healthcare delivery, advances in information sharing, the technology revolution, societal changes and development in organizational theory combine to drive the necessity of new leadership models. Expectations in the workplace, whether practice settings or academia, have shifted leadership from transactional to transformative models, emphasizing the journey of self-awareness as a central concept. Doctoral education prepares leaders concerned with analysis of the context of nursing practice, and thus, is driven by the need to provide a new generation of leaders. The emergence of transformational leadership satisfies the needs of the workers at all levels of the organization, offering meaning and purpose necessary for satisfaction and retention, outcomes that are critical for achieving the organization's mission.

References

American Hospital Association Commission on Workforce for Hospitals and Health Systems (2002). *In our hands: How hospital leaders can build a thriving workforce.* Washington, D.C.: AHA.

Bellack, J. (1999). Emotional intelligence: A missing ingredient? *Journal of Nursing Education,* **38**(1), 3–4.

Bolman, L. G. and Deal, T. E. (2001). *Leading with soul.* San Francisco. CA: Jossey-Bass.

Bolman, L. G. & Deal, T. E. (1997). *Reframing organizations: Artistry, choice, and leadership.* 2nd edn. San Francisco, CA: Jossey-Bass.

Cadman, C. and Brewer, J. (2001). Emotional intelligence: A vital prerequisite for recruitment in nursing. *Journal of Nursing Management,* **9**(6), 321–324.

Cranton, P. (1996). *Professional development as transformative learning: New perspectives for teachers of adults.* San Francisco, CA: Jossey-Bass.

Evans, D. and Allen, H. (2002). Emotional intelligence: Its role in training. *Nursing Times,* **98**(27), 41–42.

Freshwater, D. (2003). *Facilitating reflective nursing narratives in nurse education.* Paper presented at The University of Texas, Houston, November, 2003.

Freshwater, D. (2002). *Therapeutic nursing: Improving patient care through reflection.* London: Sage.

Freshwater, D., and Rolfe, G. (2001). Critical reflexivity: A politically and ethically engaged research method for nursing. *Nursing Times Research,* **6**(1), 526–537.

Freshwater, D. and Stickley, T. (in press). The heart of the art: Emotional intelligence in nurse education. *Nursing Inquiry.*

Graham, I. (2003). Leading the development of nursing within a nursing development unit: The perspectives of leadership by the team leader and a professor of nursing. *International Journal of Nursing Practice,* **9**(4), 213–222.

Grindal, D., Peterson, K., Kinneman, M. and Turner, T. (1996). The practice environment project: A process for outcome evaluation. *Journal of Nursing Administration,* **26**(5) 43–51.

Kowalski, K. and Yoder-Wise, P. (2003). Five C's of leadership. *Nurse Leader,* **1**(5), 26–31.

Jones, K., and Redman, R. (2000). Organizational culture and work redesign: experiences in three organizations. *Journal of Nursing Administration,* **30**, 604–610.

Laschinger, H. K. S., Finegan, J., Shamian, J. and Casier, S. (2000). Organizational trust and empowerment in restructured healthcare settings. *Journal of Nursing Administration,* **30**(9), 413–425.

Parker, K., Gadbois, S. (2000). Building community in the healthcare workplace. *Journal of Nursing Administration,* **30**(9), 426–431.

Porter-O'Grady, T. and Malloch, K. (2003). *Quantum leadership: A textbook of new leadership.* Boston, MA: Jones & Bartlett.

Rolfe, G., Freshwater, D. and Jasper, M. (2001). *Critical reflection for nurses and the helping professions: A user's guide.* Basingstoke: Palgrave.

Sherwood, G. D. (2003). Leadership for a healthy work environment: Caring for the human spirit. *Nurse Leader,* **1**(5), 36–40.

Sherwood, G., Thomas, E., Bennett, D., and Lewis, P. (2002). A teamwork model to improve patient safety in critical care. *Critical Care Nursing Clinics of North America,* **14**, 333–340.

Sherwood, G. (1997). Patterns of caring: the healing connection of interpersonal harmony. *International Journal for Human Caring,* **1**(1), 30–38.

Thyer, G. L. (2003). Dare to be different: Transformational leadership may hold the key to reducing the nursing shortage. *Journal of Nursing Management,* **11**(2), 73–79.

Trofino, J. (1995). Transformational leadership in health care. *Nursing Management,* **20**, 42–47.

Vitello-Cicciu, J. M. (2002). Exploring emotional intelligence: Implications for nursing leaders. *Journal of Nursing Administration,* **32**(4), 203–210.

Zemke, R., Raines, C. and Filipczak, B. (2000). *Generations at work: Managing the clash of veterans, boomers, Xers, and nexters in your workplace.* New York, NY: American Management Association.

Chapter 4

Re-envisioning the PhD Project: Implications for the preparation of future faculty in nursing

Bettina J. Woodford and Jody D. Nyquist

This chapter discusses the themes and outcomes of a national conversation in the USA focused on the state and future of doctoral education. It outlines the interrelationship of recent national calls for improvements in US doctoral education, describes the role of 'Re-envisioning the PhD Project'[1] in synthesizing those calls and in providing those who prepare and hire PhDs a set of tools for action, and offers an example of a way in which the discipline of nursing can heed the recommendations of the project to help address the current faculty shortage.

While the topic of graduate education reform is not necessarily a new one, it is being addressed today in ways that differ importantly from other times in the past. First, the exigencies of an ever-changing and increasingly complex knowledge economy, as well as labour market uncertainty, present challenges and opportunities to contemporary education unlike those experienced by earlier educators and policymakers. Secondly, the undergraduate and graduate student populations – a percentage of whom will be in the pipeline for PhD degrees, and some of whom will become our own and other nations' future professors – are becoming more diverse culturally, socioeconomically and in career orientation than ever before. A third difference is the range of voices participating in the conversation. Increasingly, leaders from business and industry, government, K-12 education (kindergarten through to 12th grade, or elementary and secondary schooling, in the USA and Canada), disciplinary associations, foundations and funding agencies, and two- and four-year colleges and universities are voicing their concerns about how well the doctoral degree helps them to meet society's educational, social, business, political and other needs. The sheer range of stakeholders is recognition that responsibility for the PhD degree is not the sole province of research universities, but more appropriately is regarded as the product of loosely structured but interdependent interactions among several different socioeconomic sectors.

In the following pages, we introduce readers to the driving forces, goals, strategies and outcomes of the Re-envisioning the PhD Project. We explain how it has served to engender and coordinate much of this national conversation, and we outline its hopes for the future of doctoral education. While focusing on the themes and recommendations for action that have emerged for doctoral education generally, we attempt to draw some important implications for nursing education specifically, particularly in the light of the nursing faculty shortage. To do so, we explore how one school of nursing, at the University of Washington, is embracing the call of re-envisioning the PhD to improve the preparation of graduate students aspiring to the nursing professoriate. Our objective is to provide doctoral educators in nursing, both in the USA and abroad, a framework for understanding their efforts to improve the doctorate in the context of this larger dialogue, to encourage them not only to learn *from* it but also to contribute their unique insights *to* it.

History and purpose of the Project

There is widespread recognition that a new, national agenda for doctoral education in the USA is emerging, motivated in part by shifts in the demand for PhDs in academic and non-academic markets and by a growing acceptance that long-held traditions in research universities must be re-examined periodically and evolve with the times.

Over the course of the 1990s, many disciplines, especially those in the arts/humanities and some social sciences, faced the threat of long-term surpluses of PhDs, while others, such as computer science, engineering and nursing, for example, faced shortfalls – particularly in relation to the numbers of PhDs choosing to remain in academe. An increasingly complex knowledge economy, coupled with labour market uncertainties, have raised questions about how well doctorate holders are prepared to apply their intellectual expertise in a range of settings where they are most likely to secure career employment. For many disciplines, the bulk of professional positions available for PhDs is not necessarily in the research universities, where only a limited number of faculty opportunities exist relative to the numbers of PhDs produced annually.

Such pragmatic concerns about the deployment of human intellectual resources catalysed several commissions and individual researchers to examine the current state of doctoral education in the USA. Recommendations for improvements have been issued by groups as diverse as the National Academy of Sciences, Committee on Science, Engineering and Public Policy (1995), the American Association of Universities (1998), the National Research Council (1998), 'The PhDs.Org Graduate School Survey' (Davis and Fiske, 1999), 'The PhDs – Ten Years Later Study' (Nerad and Cerny, 2000) and the cross-purposes report (Golde and Dore, 2000), and by several disciplinary associations. Although often very different in methodological approach, many overlapping criticisms of doctoral curricula began to emerge from these inquiries, such as potential overspecialization in research, insufficient attention to pedagogical preparation and experience, and growing disconnects in many arenas between the development of scholarly expertise and its application to pressing social and economic challenges.

What was missing from the national scene, however, was a common forum to help synthesize the multitude of recommendations for change *and* articulate opportunities for collective action. Thus, in the light of the many views of change being put forth, the goal of the Re-envisioning the PhD Project has been to stimulate a wide-reaching, active and ongoing discussion on the following question: How can we re-envision the PhD to meet the needs of society in the twenty-first century?

Developing a framework for dialogue and action

Re-envisioning the PhD draws together diverse policymakers and educators at all levels to reflect on ways of ensuring that graduate education at the modern research university will enable the PhD to thrive in the context of increasingly complex demands. The project has been driven by a philosophy of inclusion and action – inclusion of perspectives from all of the sectors of society with a stake in the processes and outcomes of PhD education, and an orientation to identifying strategies to facilitate collaborative action on ideas set forth in the national discussion.

One of our project's participants, a former dean of a comprehensive, land-grant university, succinctly captured our vision of inclusion in his opinion that a new vision of the PhD

> is a community problem. It is going to require input from federal agencies, input from industry, input from academia and from others who hire PhDs. What we have not done is sit at the same table and declare what the ground rules are going to be, because no one party can change effectively what we are trying to do.

In other words, no single level of education, type of institution, or social or academic constituency 'owns' the PhD. Instead, the doctorate should more appropriately be thought of as the product of a loose but interdependent set of relationships among those who educate PhDs, those who hire them, and those who influence the educational process. Research universities, which have a significant interest in replenishing their faculty ranks with new scholars, are not the only destination for doctorate holders. A wide range of employers, both inside and outside academe, seeks the analytical skills and problem-solving habits of mind developed in doctoral training. Academic institutions with missions primarily devoted to excellence in undergraduate learning need the PhDs they hire to have attained sufficient and high-quality instructional preparation, a solid understanding of their disciplines and the ability to navigate intellectual cross-roads with other fields of knowledge. For their part, government, not-for-profit and business and industry sectors seek candidates who understand the importance of scholarly relevance and how to apply advanced skills to national, regional and local challenges, as well as to commercial opportunities. And those who fund doctoral research and educational opportunities desire to see their investments leverage measurable benefits for groups of people beyond the individual grant recipients.

To engage as many parties as possible in the articulation of a new vision, the Re-envisioning the PhD Project conducted an environmental scan of the landscape of doctoral education, eliciting widely held concerns about the PhD and mapping the numerous innovative practices known to be emerging on campuses and in organizations. After more than 350 interviews with leaders inside and outside academe, supplemented by focus groups and e-mail surveys, nine groups of stakeholders in doctoral education emerged: doctoral students, research-intensive universities, teaching-intensive colleges and universities, K-12 education, business and industry, government funding agencies, foundations and other non-profits, disciplinary societies, and educational associations (including governance boards and accrediting bodies).

Although across these groups we noted some differences of opinion regarding the essential purposes of doctoral education, who and how many students should be admitted to doctoral study, and the model of training students should receive, we also found widespread agreement that action should be taken to address six major concerns about PhD education:

1 The time to degree needs to be shortened.
2 More ethnic and gender diversity needs to be cultivated among doctoral recipients.
3 Doctoral students need more exposure to technology, including instructional technology.
4 Doctoral students need broader professional preparation for the career opportunities available to them.
5 More global perspectives on economy, environment and culture need to be incorporated into doctoral study.
6 More opportunities for interdisciplinary work need to be fostered.

Although for the purposes of this chapter we focus, in the second half, more substantively on number four – concerns regarding professional preparation for a wide array of doctoral careers – we explore the entire array of community concerns in great detail in a project booklet entitled *Re-envisioning the PhD: What Concerns Do We Have?* (www.grad.washington.edu/envision/project_resources/concerns.html). (Nyquist and Woodford, 2000).

In April 2000, we invited some 200 leaders of these groups – those who *prepare* PhDs, those who *fund* them, those who *hire* them, and those who *influence* the doctoral enterprise in important ways, including doctoral students themselves – to participate in a national conference on re-envisioning the PhD. This forum was the first of its kind in the nation to invite several interest groups to 'sit at the same table,' as it were, to address each others' concerns and to identify multiple strategies for collaboration. A synthesis of conference themes can be found on the project's website (www.grad.washington.edu/envision/project_resources/metathemes.html) alongside the conference's proceedings, panels and sector-specific action items.

In addition to distilling community concerns and making them available to interested policymakers and educators, the project also developed several important resources to aid change agents in formulating a collective action agenda. These include:

- the national/international website itself, a living clearinghouse of transformative ideas, which is periodically updated and averages over 200,000 hits per month
- an extensive bibliography of 700+ entries addressing issues and strategies for improving doctoral education
- a collection of over 300 promising practices illustrating innovations in doctoral education from nearly 150 different institutions
- a collection of practical resources on obtaining a doctorate and on obtaining employment in diverse institutions and sectors
- an ongoing virtual discussion that extends to over 2500 stakeholders.

Issues of preparing aspiring faculty to enter a higher education system undergoing significant transformations have figured prominently in the re-envisioning project's national discussion. As Hirsch and Weber (1999) emphasize, among the many challenges universities face are those of 'providing new structures, flexible career paths and selective support for new patterns of creative inquiry, effective learning, and responsible public service' (p. 180). This range of professional endeavour requires institutions to develop multiple models of excellence (Atwell, 1996), and thus to develop faculty who are both willing and sufficiently skilled to extend themselves beyond the traditional boundaries of the lab or the lecture hall, to reach into the complex arenas of institutional governance and public scholarship, and to guide diverse learners in both the fundamental and novel applications of their disciplines.

To deal effectively with these challenges in the coming decades, doctoral students will need a kind of preparation that differs considerably from that which many of their senior faculty advisers may have acquired. Recognition of this reality is evidenced by the many promising practices being developed in universities to sharpen doctoral students' skills as innovative educators and intellectual leaders in a wide range of learning and teaching contexts (www.grad.washington.edu/envision/prom_prac.html). In the remainder of this chapter, we focus on one aspect of re-envisioning the PhD that relates specifically to enhancing the preparation of aspiring faculty, and discuss a type of collaborative strategy that may aid the nursing discipline in attracting and retaining new faculty.

The nursing faculty shortage: quantity versus quality

The current shortage of nurses and nursing faculty in the USA is a crucial issue for the recruitment *and* preparation of human and intellectual resources. It seems that more attention, however, is being paid to recruiting the desired quantity of individuals to the profession than to the quality of preparation these recruits will require to function effectively in the profession and serve as role models for attracting others. The strong focus on recruitment is understandable given the predicament of trying to increase baccalaureate enrolments in the context of a growing deficit of full-time master's and doctorally prepared faculty. Without being able to assure a sufficient number of instructors, the population of bachelor's students cannot effectively be increased. In various reports, the American Association of Colleges of Nursing (see, for example, AACN 2002, 2003a, 2003b) has been rigorously monitoring the quandary:

- Recent years have witnessed successive drops in bachelor's and master's degree enrolment nationally, along with relatively little growth in PhD programme enrolments overall.
- In response to a 2002 AACN survey of nursing schools on enrolment and graduation rates 62% pointed to faculty shortages as a reason for denying admission to numerous qualified applicants into their baccalaureate programmes.
- Replacements for a large number of anticipated faculty retirements (the mean age of current nursing faculty is 50 years) are difficult to find. Non-competitive academic salaries, the high cost and length of doctoral education, and the increasingly complex expectations of faculty performance, cause many current faculty and new PhDs to consider turning away from the academic profession.
- As much as 43% of nursing master's degree holders, and as much as 27% of doctorate holders, leave, or choose not to enter, faculty positions in the academy in order to pursue more lucrative opportunities in nursing services, the private sector or private practice.
- It is estimated that only about 50% of all faculty teaching in baccalaureate and higher degree programmes are PhD-prepared.

Proposed strategies for enlarging the recruitment pool of qualified students in the USA vary greatly, from increasing outreach to youth in K-12 education and beefing up master's programmes to targeting non-traditional groups, whether underrepresented minorities or individuals from other disciplines, to streamlining Bachelor of Science in Nursing (BSN)-to-PhD programmes, expanding distance-learning programmes, borrowing instructional time from clinicians and nurse practitioners and re-hiring retired nursing faculty to reach larger numbers of undergraduate and graduate students (Hinshaw, 2001;

AACN, 2003a). The range of creativity in these strategies is, itself, a telling indicator of the lengths to which schools of nursing find themselves going to preserve their ranks to meet the nation's challenging healthcare needs.

Of course, non-competitive salaries in academe are a major impediment to recruitment and retention of significant numbers of nursing faculty, particularly considering the opportunity costs associated with five or six or more years of expensive graduate study in addition to lost income and benefits. It is also a problem that, given the current economic slump and other factors of academic pay compared to compensation in the private sector, is not likely to be fixable in any truly effective way in the short term.

But there is another factor contributing to personnel shrinkage in the nursing professoriate, and that is the nature of the faculty career itself. Over the past 20 to 30 years, the workload demands of faculty have changed considerably, with role expectations becoming more complex and multifaceted. As Berberet and McMillin (2002) argue, today faculty members must gear up to 'secure extramural funding, conduct research, produce scholarship, offer community and university service' – all in addition to the more traditional work of teaching undergraduate and graduate students which, given the diversity of student demographics, learning styles and emerging instructional technologies, is not so traditional anymore. Maintaining clinical expertise, supervising (increasingly older) students in clinical work, and keeping fully abreast of a rapidly changing healthcare environment are additional challenges for nursing educators.

While these are not easy challenges to address, they contrast with issues of salary levels and the number of career opportunities in other sectors in that they are not numerical in nature. And this brings us to an observation: the discussions of faculty shortages in nursing revolve largely around issues of *quantity*, that is, the numbers of faculty needing to be recruited and retained in academe in order to preserve the profession's vitality. Vitality, however, is about more than increasing the numbers. Figuring less prominently in the shortage discussion is the issue of *quality*, that is, the ways in which recruits and potential recruits should best be prepared for performing a myriad of roles effectively and, therefore, for persisting – indeed thriving – in a complicated educational system. Quality is a matter of improving the performance capacity of faculty as well as fine-tuning the institutional structures in which they work.

In worrying about immediate actions that can be taken to alleviate the faculty shortage, it may be tempting to relegate quality preparation to secondary importance (however unintentionally). But quality performance is about professional development for multiple faculty roles, and insufficient role preparation constrains one's abilities to manage job stressors, leading to dissatisfaction, thereby raising the chances of leaving. Thus, quality preparation can have a direct impact on quantity. And, unlike academic salaries, professional development can begin to be improved immediately with relatively low-cost adjustments to the educational and institutional processes that produce, and maintain, nursing faculty. More students cannot be recruited effectively into nursing programmes, and ultimately into the faculty ranks, unless there is an increase in the number of faculty to teach them. Equally important, however, there must be a concomitant improvement in faculty preparedness to teach effectively and to contribute to student learning appropriately within the context of institutional mission, be it in a graduate setting or one of the more numerous, primarily undergraduate institutions.

A crucial aspect of faculty preparedness is a solid understanding of how to integrate teaching and service roles with those pertaining to research and discovery. This is not so much an issue of 'balancing' multiple roles, as if each were carried out separately but equally. Faculty development in nursing calls for a concept of preparation that successfully *interweaves* the whole range of professorial activities, such as student academic advising and career mentoring, institutional committee obligations, instructional theory, strategies and planning, curriculum design, and research, writing and publishing, among others. The AACN has recognized that a broader definition of nursing scholarship, to include the activities associated with teaching and learning as part of the full range of intellectual responsibilities within the discipline of nursing, will aid doctoral programmes in aligning curricula to support a notion of scholarly practice better suited to meeting contemporary knowledge demands (AACN, 1999).

Similarly, the National League for Nursing (NLN), in a 2002 position statement, stipulates that quality education of new generations of nurses and future nursing professors hinges on faculty who 'understand their role, can implement that role effectively, and can influence the future of nursing education.' To highlight the importance of preparation for the faculty role, the NLN's statement draws an analogy between the knowledge and skill needed to treat patients properly and that needed to support student learning successfully:

> We in nursing would never think of allowing an individual to practice as a nurse practitioner if she or he did not have a sound knowledge base and highly developed skills in assessment, diagnosis, pharmacotherapeutics, reimbursement issues, parameters of the role, and so on. Yet we constantly allow individuals to practice as teachers with no or only cursory knowledge of, and skill in, teaching, advisement, curriculum design, program evaluation, outcomes assessment, accreditation processes, citizenship in the academic community, principles of higher education, evaluation strategies, and so on. This must change.
>
> (Valiga, 2002, p. 3)

In much the same way as effective and talented nurses generate appreciation for the profession by helping people to improve their health, truly effective preparation will enable faculty to be excited about and dedicated to their challenging work, and thus better able to serve students' diverse learning needs as well as inspire students to see this crucial institutional role as a viable, attractive career option in which to exercise their professional leadership in nursing science, education and practice. We do not mean to imply that improved professional development alone is a cure-all for securing the 40,000 individuals that potentially will be needed in the nursing education enterprise before the end of this decade (NLN, 2002).[2] On the other hand, there is no doubt that high-quality, comprehensive preparation is critical for preparing professors to be role models for successive generations of potential nursing entrants. While many nursing leaders in universities and policy organizations are posing the question, Will there be enough faculty to teach our future nursing students? It is equally indispensable to ask, *How well* will those faculty recruited be able to teach, and guide the disciplinary and career development of future students? How can we ensure that nursing educators acquire the tools they will need to confidently thrive in the profession and, despite all the system's imperfections, stick with it? In this context of nursing's immediate and long-term future needs, it seems instructive to ask a simple question: Is improved professional development for challenging faculty roles an expendable commodity?

Even if we answer that last question with a resounding 'No', we must acknowledge that faculty development does not begin with newly appointed faculty. It begins much earlier in the pipeline, during what has been called the anticipatory socialization stage of professional development (van Maanen, 1976). During doctoral study, students commence a learning and emulation period in which they begin to assume the values, attitudes and behaviours of the intellectual profession they wish to join (Bess, 1978; Austin, 2002). While not every doctoral student intends to pursue a faculty career, it is in this stage where rigorous exposure to the many sides of the profession, including but not limited to research, is crucial in providing aspiring faculty the tools they need to carry out their goals, and in inspiring potential recruits to seriously consider the faculty pathway.

Most researchers of graduate student development agree that, while leaving room for some disciplinary variation, the vast majority of doctoral students, including those who aspire to faculty appointments, enter their degree programmes with poorly formed ideas about what it means to become a faculty member. Sometimes rather than provide clarity, PhD programmes inadvertently make the picture murkier for even the brightest of students. During doctoral programmes, many students grapple with mixed messages about the relationship between teaching, research and service; receive unsystematic, if any real, mentoring; and find it difficult to access concrete information about career prospects, and the multiple facets of faculty roles, especially regarding the differences between teaching in research universities and in other types of colleges and universities (where the majority of faculty positions are located) (Nyquist et al, 1999). These problems are in no way the result of ill will on the part of faculty, but rather, a manifestation of deeper drivers of institutional behaviour, such as research funding policies and an institutional prestige culture that values research over education, knowledge production over knowledge transmission, and 'doing things the way they have always been done' over doing what makes most sense given the inescapable evolution of our educational reality. In this context, faculty are often underprepared to offer doctoral students the systematic feedback, close mentoring and overall career development guidance they need to make informed decisions about their professional futures. To the extent that this situation also applies to the nursing discipline, it is not difficult to imagine that some students develop less-than-desirable images of faculty life and proceed to seek career options in other pastures, sometimes even before completing the PhD.

There is also widespread agreement that the graduate education process can, and is well positioned to, do much more to make graduate student professional development less haphazard. As noted earlier, one of the primary purposes of the Re-envisioning the PhD Project has been to learn about, and provide all graduate educators access to, the hundreds of promising practices being implemented around the country and abroad to address such concerns, particularly as they relate to the development and deployment of aspiring faculty. In most cases, innovations in graduate education do not require major influxes of new funds, but can be carried out successfully with minimal investments, as long as these are coupled with structural improvements in the graduate curriculum and with effective engagement of resource partners within and/or outside of the university who can aid, as well as benefit from, a graduate process that is more responsive to doctoral students' and their potential employers' needs.

One such innovation involves broadening the traditional doctoral student experience by providing aspiring faculty direct exposure to the range of ways effective faculty members, in a variety of educational settings, manage their research, pedagogical and institutional roles and responsibilities. The Preparing Future Faculty programme (PFF), initiated by the American Association of Colleges and Universities and the Council of Graduate Schools (www.preparing-faculty.org), pioneered a professional preparation concept intended to help doctoral programmes in all disciplines more effectively integrate the development of teaching and governance competencies with the research competencies of PhD students. Numerous doctoral institutions in the USA have participated in the programme, including several nursing programmes, while many others have created their own, home-grown versions (www.preparing-faculty.org/PFFWeb.like.htm).

The experience students undergo, usually involving some combination of specially designed seminars, organized sessions with alumni who have become successful faculty, visits to other campuses, shadowing a professor, and in some cases, a teaching internship with a professor in one's own university or another institution, is deeper and wider than the traditional teaching assistantship. That is because at the heart of this concept is a resource partnership, wherein the research-doctoral institution encourages participating departments to forge relationships with their disciplinary colleagues in nearby liberal arts colleges, four-year institutions, comprehensive universities or community colleges. These institutions, whose missions emphasize excellence in teaching large numbers of undergraduate students, help the graduate programme to extend the kind of classroom and professional development experience that its doctoral students need, while also helping the research university educate itself about what is needed to construct a model of preparation that more broadly prepares future faculty to thrive in diverse educational settings. In turn, the partner college gains a more active voice in shaping the preparation of the kinds of faculty it would like to hire, and provides its own faculty, who commonly do not have their own graduate students, a unique opportunity for dynamic professional stimulation with advanced doctoral students and graduate faculty. Doctoral students gain a dedicated faculty mentor and intimate involvement with multiple faculty responsibilities, ranging from curriculum design, programme planning, teaching diverse students (often with new learning technologies) and the workings of faculty meetings and initiatives. The duration of the student's experience, which often can be undertaken for credit, typically ranges from one or two quarters to an academic year.

A case of re-envisioning the PhD in nursing

Having participated in the Re-envisioning the PhD 2000 National Conference, the Dean of the School of Nursing at the University of Washington (UW) and its nursing faculty have been asking the question, How can we re-envision nursing doctoral education to meet the pressing educational needs of the Pacific Northwest region and the nation?[3] As the highest-ranked nursing programme in the USA, the School is committed to continually seeking innovative ways for its graduate students to excel in the field's diverse pathways.

Since that conference, the School of Nursing has begun developing an agenda of innovation in the doctoral core curriculum and in PhD student professional development. First, by participating in the Preparing Future Faculty programme in 2001, under the auspices of the UW Graduate School, the nursing programme was able to have two doctoral students engage in teaching internships with faculty colleagues at UW's two branch campuses. The initial outcomes have been enlightening, both for students and for the School of Nursing itself.

One of the students reported several benefits that otherwise would have been extremely difficult to obtain without her teaching internship.[4] First, she discovered that the integration of research and teaching is not an elusive, abstract goal, but indeed a tangible, attainable one and beneficial to her performance as a doctoral student and potential faculty member. A partnership with a master teacher, who offers courses in aging and dying, allowed this PFF participant to put her doctoral research on end-of-life care to work in the service of undergraduate pedagogy. In agreement with the master teacher, she not only spent regular time observing and assisting with instruction, but took over responsibility for delivering several modules of the course. With assistance from her mentor, and with supplemental consultations at the UW Center for Instructional Development & Research, she infused the modules with her own content knowledge by adapting concepts and findings from her own research to explanations, materials and exercises appropriate to learning at the undergraduate level.

In addition to direct classroom experience, hours spent in mentoring discussions with this faculty member helped the mentee to understand how professors at teaching-intensive institutions effectively handle a heavy course load (much heavier than her own research professors) and the tools needed to balance those responsibilities with significant commitments to committee work and other kinds of institutional priorities. Animated and dynamic discussions about how to address diverse students' learning styles, the more applied and immediate professional concerns of (older) Bachelor's students in the branch campus, and how to navigate departmental politics, became the preferred topics of the hour-long car commute the mentee and mentor enjoyed together several times a week. This level of pedagogical and career-oriented involvement in her professional development would be, the mentee believed, more difficult to obtain in her doctoral programme, where the focus of discussions more commonly revolves around research.

A short time after completing her internship, the branch campus invited this PhD student to be the sole instructor of record for another nursing course. To date she has served the branch campus in that capacity for an additional two quarters, expanding significantly the original benefit of the PFF internship to her professional development, to the host institution and to its nursing students.

Perhaps one of the most heartening observations this mentee offered about the value of her internship experience was that no other component of her graduate education had allowed her to realize just how much she enjoyed teaching, both as an intellectual and professional endeavour. She went on to reveal how her perspectives on instruction and learning, which she described as relatively narrow prior to working with her mentor, had not only expanded but now were more substantively informing her plans for securing a faculty position upon graduation, even though earlier in her education the idea of working in a policy think-tank had been an inspiration for graduate school.

In part inspired by the high level of student interest shown when the two teaching internships were originally advertised, the School of Nursing began to consider other ways to enhance the doctoral curriculum. In 2002, a faculty task force was formed to identify ways to meet the School's goal of increasing enrolment in the doctoral programme by making it attractive to more candidates, and graduating more nursing educators. Key to these considerations is revising the core curriculum to integrate more educationally, clinically and organizationally focused emphases. A core curriculum category of Theory and Domain of Knowledge might be revised in the future to include two courses, one on pedagogical practices in nursing education, and one on curriculum development. In addition, courses in the UW College of Education also might be designated for several credits of independent nursing study (e.g. perspectives on educational leadership, special topics in higher education, dynamics of educational organizations, etc.).

Also under consideration are ways to offer doctoral students more teaching assistantships, either for remuneration or for special credit or both, the latter consisting of a special seminar in pedagogical issues in combination with some form of assistance to a nursing school professor or an instructional project. Currently, the availability of national funds for Preparing Future Faculty is uncertain, but many universities that have benefited from the programme are seeking ways to mobilize local resources with their partners to continue offering these important experiences to their doctoral students. The fortunate geographical situation of the UW School of Nursing is conducive to considering multilateral agreements with a range of two- and four-year colleges in the Puget Sound region to generate self-sustaining means and novel ways for those who produce future faculty and those who desperately need them to partner in the process.

Conclusion

This chapter has outlined the interrelationship of recent national calls for improvements in US doctoral education, described the role of Re-envisioning the PhD Project in synthesizing those calls and in providing those who prepare and hire PhDs a set of tools for action, and offered one example of a way in which the discipline of nursing can heed the recommendations to alleviate the current faculty shortage.

At present, it is not yet known whether these possible adjustments in the UW nursing doctoral curriculum indeed will help significantly to boost enrolment and retention of aspiring future faculty. Nonetheless, the educational re-emphasis is a strong sign of the current faculty's recognition that 'virtually all [our] doctoral students will go on to teach [in academe or outside it], yet we do not explicitly prepare them for this future' (unofficial planning document, 2003). Such acknowledgement constitutes an important step in revising and realigning doctoral study to support critical needs in the preparation and maintenance of excellent aspiring nursing faculty. It is also a sign of the School's responsiveness to the faculty shortage regionally and nationally, in such a way that meaningful experiences of, and knowledge about, the wide-ranging roles and responsibilities of nursing faculty can be more smoothly integrated into the core curriculum. Curricular integration is a strategy recommended by virtually all the national studies on improving doctoral education, which advocate not designating such opportunities as add-ons or leaving them up to the whims of chance exposure. Although the Re-envisioning the PhD Project outlined several areas of needed action, we can definitely emphasize that in terms of the critical shortage of nursing faculty, the future is now. We look forward to following the UW School of Nursing's successes in embracing that future.

Notes

1 This project was supported by a grant from the Pew Charitable Trusts and by the Graduate School of the University of Washington. The opinions expressed in this chapter are those of the authors and do not necessarily reflect those of the funding organizations.

2 The article's calculations rely on the following assumptions. Approximately 3500 nursing programmes currently house approximately 300,000 students. Enrolments may need to increase by a third to meet the projected shortfall of nurses in the USA, bringing the desired number of total enrolments to 400,000. At an ideal ratio of 10:1 (students:full-time faculty member), 40,000 faculty would need to be in place, of which currently there is less than half.

3 We thank Dean Nancy Fugate Woods, Associate Dean Susan Woods, Professor David Allen and doctoral student Jamie Goldstein-Shirley for sharing with us how the School of Nursing has been pursuing ways to implement re-envisioning strategies in its preparation of aspiring nursing faculty.

4 A second Preparing Future Faculty doctoral student participant was unavailable for comment.

References

American Association of Colleges of Nursing (1999). Defining scholarship for the discipline of nursing. (Position statement). Washington, DC: American Association of Colleges of Nursing. Available at: http://www.aacn.nche.edu/Publications/positions/scholar.htm (accessed on 19.05.04).

AACN (2002). *Faculty resignations and retirements.* (Unpublished data). Washington, DC: American Association of Colleges of Nursing.

AACN (2003a). *Faculty shortages in baccalaureate and graduate nursing programs: Scope of the problem and strategies for expanding the supply.* (White paper). Washington, DC: American Association of Colleges of Nursing. Available at http://www.aacn.nche.edu/Publications/WhitePapers/FacultyShortages.htm (accessed on 19.05.04).

AACN (2003b). *2002–2003 Enrollment and graduations in baccalaureate and graduate programs in nursing*. Washington, DC: American Association of Colleges of Nursing.

American Association of Universities (1998). *Committee on Graduate Education: Report and recommendations*. Available at http://www.aau.edu/reports/GradEdRpt.pdf (accessed on 19.05.04).

Atwell, R. (1996). Doctoral education must match needs and realities. *Chronicle of Higher Education,* 43(14). Available at: http://chronicle.com/data/articles.dir/art-43.dir/issue-14.dir/14b00401.htm (accessed on 20.05.04).

Austin, A. (2002). Preparing the next generation of faculty: Graduate school as socialization to the academic career. *Journal of Higher Education,* 73(1), 94–122.

Berberet, J. and McMillin, L. (2002). The American professoriate in transition. *AGB Priorities*, Spring (18), 1–15. Washington, DC: Association of Governing Boards of Universities and Colleges.

Bess, J. (1978). Anticipatory socialization of graduate students. *Research in Higher Education,* 8, 289–317.

Davis, G. and Fiske, P. (1999). The PhDs.Org Graduate School Survey report of results. Available at: http://nextwave.sciencemag.org/cgi/content/full/1999/11/11/14. (accessed 20.05.04).

Golde, C.M. and Dore, T.M. (2001). *At cross-purposes: What the experiences of today's doctoral students reveal about doctoral education.* Wisconsin Center for Education Research. Available at: http://www.phd-survey.org (accessed on 19.05.04).

Hinshaw, A. S. (2001). A continuing challenge: The shortage of educationally prepared nursing faculty. *Online Journal of Issues in Nursing.* **6**(1). Available at: http://www.nursingworld.org/ojin/topic14/tpc14_3.htm (accessed on 15.08.03).

Hirsch, W. and Weber, L. (eds) (1999). *Challenges facing higher education at the millennium.* Phoenix, AZ: Oryx Press.

National Academy of Sciences, Committee on Science, Engineering, and Public Policy (1995). *Reshaping the graduate education of scientists and engineers.* Washington, DC: National Academy Press. Available at: http://books.nap.edu/catalog/4935.html (accessed on 11.07.03).

National League for Nursing (2002). Position statement: The preparation of nurse educators. *Nursing Education Perspectives,* **23**(5), 267–269.

National Research Council (1998). *Trends in the early careers of life scientists.* Washington, DC: National Academy Press. Available at: http://books.nap.edu/catalog/6244.html (accessed on 15.08.03).

Nerad, M. and Cerny, J. (2000). Improving doctoral education: Recommendations from the PhDs – Ten Years Later Study. *The Council of Graduate Schools Communicator,* **33**(2), 6.

Nyquist, J. and Woodford, B. (2000). *Re-envisioning the PhD: What concerns do we have?* Seattle, WA: Center for Instructional Development & Research and the Graduate School, University of Washington.

Nyquist, J., Manning, L., Wulff, D. et al. (1999). On the road to becoming a professor: The graduate student experience. *Change Magazine*, pp. 18–27. Available at: http://www.grad.washington.edu/envision/resources/road.html (accessed on 11.07.03).

Valiga, T. (2002). *The nursing faculty shortage: National League for Nursing perspective.* Presentation given to the National Advisory Council on Nurse Education and Practice. Available at: http://www.nln.org/slides/speach.htm. (accessed on 15.08.03).

Van Maanen, J. (1976). Breaking in: Socialization to work. In: R. Dubin (ed). *Handbook of work, organizations and society.* Chicago, IL: Rand-McNally College Publishing, pp. 67–130.

Chapter 5

Doctoral education in nursing: opportunities and dynamics in the marketplace

Richard W. Redman and Lynn Chenoweth

Recent decades have been characterized by continual, transformational changes on a global level, a phenomenon particularly evident in healthcare. The changes in the delivery of healthcare services have affected both the practice and the education of all health professionals, especially for nurses. The changing needs of contemporary society, and nursing's response to these, have resulted in a rapid expansion of nursing education, particularly in the university setting, and a demand for a variety of advanced practice and leadership opportunities.

This chapter examines the impact of these changes on the demands for nurses with advanced preparation at the doctoral level. While doctoral preparation has typically been seen as the pathway for a career in academe, the needs and dynamics in society have challenged this tradition in ways that could not have been anticipated 30 years ago. More recently, doctoral education, in nursing as in all disciplines, has received close examination in terms of the pressing needs of society and the deficiencies in doctoral programmes in meeting these needs. The supply of and demand for doctorally prepared nurses varies considerably as do the pathways that nurses take for doctoral preparation. The challenges of stakeholder needs and global forces, which present challenges to both the discipline and educational institutions, will also be examined. Case studies of doctorally prepared nurses are described to profile the different pathways and career trajectories that might be found in various settings. Finally, an agenda for present and future needs is presented.

Doctoral education: the traditional view

Graduate education in all disciplines is undergoing rapid change as a reflection of changing social dynamics. In the USA, the original vision for graduate education was to train scholars for the transmission and creation of knowledge. Most US universities based their approaches to graduate education on the German model of education, emphasizing the generation of new knowledge. In the latter part of the twentieth century, however, the broad goals of doctoral education began to change, expanding beyond the expectations for generation of scientific knowledge through research and scholarly activities, to meeting the needs of society through leadership roles in a variety of settings.

In nursing doctoral education, two prevailing models for curriculum have evolved. These have been described as the European model and the North American model (Ketefian and Redman, 2001). Both of these models focus on advanced preparation in the discipline of nursing. In general, the purpose of these programmes is to prepare scientists who are qualified to develop and test nursing knowledge and leaders who will assume positions in education or the healthcare delivery system. In the European model, there generally is no or little formal coursework and the programme is conducted through individually supervised research. In the North American model, there is extensive coursework, generally for one to two years, followed by comprehensive examinations and independent research culminating in the dissertation. Variations of these now are found in several areas of the world (Ketefian et al, 2001; McKenna and Cutcliffe, 2001). Many disciplines, such as education, business and public health, have developed professional doctorates. Others, such as psychology, developed clinical doctorates. Nursing has followed this trend although there is no clear agreement as yet on the best approach. In Australia the professional nursing doctorate has adopted the North American PhD model.

In nursing, many programmes in the USA do not differentiate much in programme goals or curricula, even though the degrees that are conferred may vary. Nor is there evidence that prospective students make a deliberate choice for graduate study based on the type of degree offered (Redman and Ketefian, 1997). However, this broadening of the purposes of graduate study and the opportunities available for doctorally prepared graduates is evident in society today.

Internationally, nurses have responded to global changes in healthcare delivery in different ways. One response has been the further development of nurses' educational preparation for practice and leadership. Williams (1996) described this need and urged African-American nurses to act on change through re-education, in order to pioneer relevant and effective health outcomes for clients and their families. At the present time the nursing profession, as do all health professions, demands evidence-based, outcome-driven care interventions, whatever the context of care. The discovery of new knowledge, rapidly changing social expectations and uncertainty within social structures, call for a critical review of nursing knowledge and skills. Continuing education, therefore, is an essential process at this time of national and global change (Bazely, 2003).

Career pathways for the doctorally prepared nurse

While it is assumed that once a doctorate is obtained, the graduates will spend their career in academe, teaching and conducting research, that is not always the case. Some do not find academe an attractive career pathway due to non-competitive salaries, the general demands of a faculty position, and the struggles to maintain both family and a research career (Fogg, 2003). Limited data exist but what is available indicate a variety of career options that might be chosen (Committee on Dimensions, Causes and Implications of Recent Trends in the Careers of Life Scientists, 1998).

Table 5.1 presents recent data on the employment commitments of doctoral graduates in the USA and Australia. In all disciplines, employment in institutions of higher education was only slightly higher than 50%. This is somewhat misleading in the USA in that an additional 29% entered into postdoctoral fellowships which, for the most part, are carried out in university settings. What is surprising, however, is the fact that a number of graduates entered positions in industry or the policy arena.

The comparable data for nursing doctoral graduates are also presented. While a larger number of nursing graduates become employed in educational institutions, the overall total is actually lower because far fewer nursing graduates enter into postdoctoral fellowships. Approximately 22% of nursing graduates in the USA and 49% in Australia assume non-academic positions in clinical research or practice, executive level administration, consultation and the policy arena. Comparative data for other countries are not available. However, the limited data in Table 5.1 indicate differences in the two major systems and this suggests patterns that would likely vary in other countries as well.

Supply and demand issues

While large numbers of doctoral graduates do enter academic positions after graduation, the supply and demand issues vary across disciplines. For example, in the USA, there is a growing shortage of faculty in nursing programmes and enrolments of qualified students are being affected because of this (Berlin and Sechrist, 2002; American Association of Colleges of Nursing [AACN], 2003). This critical shortage of nursing faculty is due to a number of factors including aging of the current faculty with insufficient numbers of younger faculty to replace them, the unattractiveness of an academic career for new doctoral graduates and the lack of competitive salaries in academic settings when compared with the healthcare services sector or industry.

The US Bureau of Labor Statistics (cited in Phillips, 1998, p. 493) reveals that interest in research careers outside of the university system is appealing to many doctoral graduates, particularly in government departments and healthcare services as managers and administrators (Wolff, 1995; Taylor and Hardy, 1996; Smallwood, 2001). Industry and business are absorbing those with an interest outside of the traditional academic role, along with globalization of health goods, services and research, and the higher salaries offered outside of academia (Golde and Fiske, 2000; Smallwood, 2001). For example, while the demand for postdoctoral science and psychology positions has traditionally been high, many doctoral students perceive that broadening their career horizons creates

Table 5.1 Employment commitment of graduates upon graduation from doctoral programmes in the USA and Australia, 2001–2002.

	USA		*Australia*	
	All Disciplines[a]	*Nursing*[b]	*All Disciplines*[c]	*Nursing*[c]
Number of doctoral degrees awarded	41,368	457	28,632	49
Definite employment commitment after graduation	71.1%	98%	Unavailable	100% all responses
No employment commitment	28.9%	2%	Unavailable	Nil
Employment in institutions of higher education	51.8%	68.8%	Unavailable	51%
Policy arena: governmental agency	8.4%	1.3%		1.0%
Postdoctoral study	28.9%	3.9%		1.0%
Employment in industry or self-employment	21.1%	22.5%	Unavailable	49%
Nursing only				
Clinical research/ practice		10.7%		45%
Executive level administration		8.5%		1.0%
Consultation		1.3%		1.0%
Military		1.0%		Unavailable
Business or industry		1.0%		Unavailable

Notes

a Estimates are from annual survey in the USA (*Doctoral Recipients from United States Universities: Summary Report 2001*) and cover the entire year, 2001. Some entries result in dual counting and thus, the total exceeds 100%. See Hoffer et al (2001).

b Estimates are from American Association of Colleges of Nursing, *Enrollment and Graduations in Baccalaureate and Graduate Programs in Nursing, 2001–2002*, and cover the year from August 2001–July 2002. Note that 3.5% of graduates are unaccounted for in these data.

c *Higher Education Students Time Series Tables 2001 Graduate Destination Survey*. Department of Employment, Education and Training, Australia.

more employment opportunities and options, given the fluctuating funding of academic and university research positions over time (Zimpfer and DeTrude, 1990; Golde and Fiske, 2000).

The international nursing marketplace seeks nurses who can provide new types of services in ways not previously considered. Doctorally prepared nurses are creating opportunities to advance nursing scholarship, research and leadership, and are also contributing significantly to crafting social policy and setting the healthcare agenda (Horn, 1999). Exciting entrepreneurial opportunities presented themselves in the 1990s in the form of private healthcare agencies and consultancy services (Williams, 1996). This shows that employers from a wide range of areas are interested in hiring PhDs (Horn, 1999), although the increasing number of doctoral graduates worldwide has attracted some criticism (see for example, Atwell, 1996). Given the relatively fewer numbers of nurses graduating with either PhDs or professional doctorates, their potential career horizon is limitless. These career opportunities may or may not have been considered by students during the doctoral journey itself.

Like most other health science students wishing to undertake higher degrees in their field, nurses have traditionally considered the doctorate as training for careers in academic and research fields (La Pidus, 1995; Magner, 1998; Horn, 1999; Moyer and Salovey, 1999). The role of training through research is crucial in gaining this career path for doctoral graduates. Indeed, many disciplines describe doctoral training as a process of cooptation by peers (Deneef, 2000; Mangematin et al, 2000). While the current figures on the percentages of graduating Australian nurses opting for academic careers are limited to responses on the Australian Universities Graduate Survey, approximately half choose academic careers. In countries where nursing education has been transferred to the tertiary education system over the past few decades, this trend is common (see, for example, Smith et al, 2000). However, in countries like the USA, with a longer tradition of higher education in nursing, the career options for the doctoral graduate are broad, in line with career expectations (Moyer and Salovey, 1999). So far as research careers are concerned in the USA and UK, the US National Academy of Sciences (NAS) and the UK National Science Foundation (NSF) claim that only one third of those receiving doctorates expect to enter the academic tenure system (Phillips, 1998).

While fluctuations in market demand and supply have occurred for doctoral graduates in many disciplines since the early 1980s, this is not generally the case for nursing (Williams, 1996). Nevertheless, given the increasing influence of world events on national job markets, all graduates are urged to maintain a degree of flexibility when searching for employment and making career choices (Deneef, 2000; McGinn, 2000; Smallwood, 2001). Mangematin et al (2000) point out that a doctoral degree, unlike a coursework master's degree, must comprise an essential component of a career plan, rather than be regarded as an automatic stepping-stone for gaining employment. For example, the academic market for health-related doctorates between 1986 and 1992 was far less than that for engineering, science and political science graduates, even though the number of graduates was small (Cheng and Davidson, 2001). This is explained by the 'cobweb model' of supply and demand, whereby the escalation of high market demand and wage prospects for doctoral graduates during the years they are studying begin to wane when the market becomes saturated with new graduates. These periods of 'boom and bust' are related to the lag time in the education process, a situation relevant to any doctoral graduate (Cheng and Davidson, 2001).

Another cause of disappointment for graduates in the job market is potential discrepancy between the employer's expectations and the student's educational training. If an employer is not looking primarily for a researcher skilled in a particular methodology with deep knowledge of a particular field of inquiry, but rather a skilled problem solver, team leader and catalyst for change, the doctoral graduate may need further experiential learning to meet the job requirements (Mangematin et al, 2000). This has traditionally been the case for graduates of counselling (Zimpfer and DeTrude, 1990), chemistry (Brennan, 1997), political science and politics (Yin, 1998), and in the life sciences, behavioural and social sciences and in education (Malveaux, 1995). In more recent years career options of female graduates have been hampered by employer expectations combined with the pressure of family commitments, such as an expectation that private time be employed to publish, family-unfriendly workplaces and tokenistic equal employment opportunities (Moyer and Salovey, 1999). While many doctoral graduates seek employment in prestigious university posts, these are often limited to those achieving high grades and/or those who have maintained part-time employment within the academic department or faculty during their candidature (Xiao, 2000).

Changing perspectives on doctoral education

The overall approach to doctoral education has come under increasing scrutiny in the past five years, particularly but not exclusively in the USA. Often, employers of doctoral graduates are critical of the lack of various skills in the graduates vis-à-vis needs of the contemporary workplace. Some of the criticism around doctoral education has focused on how the curriculum and learning experiences prepare 'citizen scholars' who can better meet the needs of society (Nyquist, 2002). These criticisms have examined graduates in faculty and non-academic positions alike. Because of these issues, innovations and alternative models for doctoral programmes are beginning to appear in universities.

The types of skills that all employers are looking for today have several common themes. Employers in all types of settings value the research skills and ability to think critically that are typically found in doctoral graduates. However, these employers also need doctoral graduates with the ability to function in teams, conduct committee meetings and facilitate decision making in a group context, the ability to manage conflict and create productive work environments with other employees who come from increasingly diverse backgrounds and points of view, and to work in environments that are continually changing. Current critics find the learning experiences in many doctoral programmes too intense and narrow, too lengthy, focused primarily on research training and knowledge generation without a requirement for application of that knowledge to address contemporary social issues, too discipline- and campus-based with insufficient learning experiences in the community, and insufficient preparation of doctoral graduates to assume leadership positions (Cherwitz and Sullivan, 2002; Gaff, 2002; Nyquist and Woodford, 2002).

A major project, entitled 'Re-envisioning the PhD', has been examining the issues from the perspectives of various stakeholders of doctoral education programmes (see Chapter 4). These stakeholders include faculty, funding agencies, leaders in industry and the public policy arena, and students themselves. Interviews from over 400 stakeholders have produced the development of a variety of core competencies for doctoral graduates to be successful in assuming leadership roles in the academic, government, and the non-profit and corporate sectors. In addition to disciplinary knowledge, these competencies include teaching competency, understanding diversity, an ability to connect one's work with that of others across disciplines, a global perspective and an ability to understand ethical conduct in a social context (Nyquist, 2002).

Market demands

Many academics argue that doctoral education must match the needs of the nation (see, for example, Randolph, 1990; Atwell, 1996; Phillips, 1998; McGinn, 2000). Faculty shortages of doctorally prepared nurses in the USA are growing steadily. Demand has exceeded supply and this is expected to continue for the foreseeable future (AACN, 2002; Berlin et al, 2003). LaPidus (1996) argues that graduates must know their fields, understand the process of scholarly inquiry and realistically grasp how these valuable skills may be deployed across a variety of purposes, settings and careers. In the field of science, industry is looking for highly trained individuals with good technical grounding, excellent writing skills, an understanding of statistics, computing and often mathematical skills, ability to undertake a variety of research processes, and effective interpersonal skills (Phillips, 1998; Golde and Fiske, 2000). Whatever the field, the propensity for working independently and effectively under pressure, particularly to solve problems in variable conditions, is another key factor in securing employment (Mangematin et al, 2000; Hertel et al, 2001).

These qualities are most likely to be identified in students undertaking part-time employment or apprenticeships in industry during their studies. Securing a university scholarship or grant, thereby negating the necessity to seek work in industry during candidature, greatly reduces the probability of finding a permanent position in industry upon graduating (Mangematin et al, 2000). For example, Zimpfer and DeTrude (1990) identified that while counselling graduates were highly job mobile, 41.7% were able to return to their industry-based positions and the remainder were highly sought after in the private market because of their ability to apply their knowledge and problem-solving skills to the position.

The potential for an academic appointment rests largely with success as a student in many countries (Phillips, 1998; Mangematin et al, 2000). Top ranking universities continue to hire highly achieving graduates, whereas less competitive universities are keen to establish relationships with industries for linked research projects (Horn, 1999). Securing a research grant for doctoral studies, publishing and securing part-time work during candidature, being supervised by highly regarded academics and undertaking the degree at a prestigious university, completing the degree on time and achieving high grades during study, are the hallmarks of a successful student who seeks an academic career. However, these student outcomes apply more to research than to teaching careers in academe, and having a temporary or part-time academic position prior to or during the candidature is more likely to provide teaching opportunities for the graduate. Recruitment prospects can also depend on the reputation or visibility of the university, the reputation of its members, and hence, its funding capacity (Mangematin et al, 2000).

Social issues: benefits and costs

The current push for doctoral students in all fields of inquiry, and the training opportunities available to them are both problematic issues. There are social costs in undertaking doctoral studies (Wolff, 1995; LaPidus, 1997; Phillips, 1998; Yin, 1998; McGinn, 2000). Atwell (1996) argues that most new doctoral graduates are weighted down by debt and insecurity about their futures. The necessity for many doctoral students to undertake part-time studies in order to support themselves and their families with part-time work, thereby extending the candidature over five years or more, has several social consequences. If employment opportunities are not commensurate with graduate expectations, they may be forced to seek positions at their previous levels of employment, or in completely new fields or locations, or be forced to take part-time employment at a lower salary than previously if they have not been able to maintain employment links with their previous employer (Phillips, 1998; Moyer and Salovey, 1999; Hult, 2000; Xiao, 2000). The personal cost to graduates and their families is high in these situations. This issue highlights the contradictions which exist between the current educational system and the dynamic market economy.

The consequence of not being trained adequately in applied research during doctoral study is also a problem for many graduates and one of the reasons for failing to find desired employment in the marketplace (Mangematin et al, 2000). In fields where the number of graduates is relatively small, for example in nursing (Williams, 1996) and political science or politics (Yin, 1998), degree status continues to be the best indicator for employment, as it does in countries with few doctoral programmes such as in China (Xiao, 2000). Only the most highly achieving graduates or those guaranteed employment upon graduation are likely to benefit from their degrees in the short term (Hult, 2000; Xiao, 2000; Golde and Fiske, 2000). Many will return to previously held positions at the same salary, despite greater expectations placed on them (McGinn, 2000), or undertake positions which do not allow them to use their advanced knowledge and skills at a commensurate level (Siegfried and Stock, 1999).

Many graduates, therefore, are unable to contribute to their field of inquiry through further research, scholarship and teaching (Atwell, 1996; Lieberman, 1997; Smallwood, 2001). Less prestigious universities are responding to this challenge by preparing their students for applied research, rather than academic careers. The graduate's ability to work on an array of problems is promoted over specialization in accord with many employers' requirements (Horn, 1999). However, the most prestigious universities and faculties are not heeding market drivers, and the skills of research and teaching which could contribute to the faculty's continued growth are increasingly being lost to industry and the corporate world (Smallwood, 2001).

A seldom discussed social cost is the attrition of students from doctoral programmes. About 50% of those who begin work towards a doctoral degree never finish. This high attrition rate is described as 'one of academe's best kept secrets.' In nursing the attrition rate is much lower, but the concerns are similar to those expressed in the literature. The attrition rate for women and racial/ethnic minorities is even higher but exact figures are not known (Delamont et al, 2000; Lovitts, 2001). The high attrition rates are due to multiple factors: disillusionment with the academic role, the absence of strong mentoring, disappointment with the learning experience, personal life circumstances. The costs to the students who leave, as well as to the universities and society for their partial investment in the students, have not been calculated but are likely substantial.

Case studies

The view that doctoral training can result in various career pathways is presented in two case studies in the Exhibit section in this chapter. The expectation for careers in academe and/or research is borne out in one of the cases. The potential for conducting research and generating new knowledge, supervising the research work of others, and serving in leadership positions that contribute to senior management agendas is a realistic aspiration for the doctoral graduate. These career plans may be achieved through a range of avenues as unique opportunities become available. While the opportunities and the avenues of preparation will vary from country to country, the potential positions seem limited only by the interests and motivation of the doctorally prepared nurses.

Agenda for nursing education

The issues and challenges in doctoral education in general, and nursing in particular, seem to have some universal themes. While the educational approaches and opportunities will vary in different educational and social systems, there appears to be a common agenda that could be addressed globally for the benefit of nursing and healthcare. The critical next steps offered for consideration are as follows:

1. *Development of a global database for doctoral nursing education.* While there is a comprehensive listing of nursing doctoral education programmes internationally, developed and maintained by the International Network for Doctoral Education in Nursing (INDEN, 2003), there are very limited data available on the number of graduates produced by these programmes, the variety of curricular approaches employed, and the types of positions that graduates fulfil. Data on the number of graduates and their postgraduation positions vary considerably throughout the international community. These types of data are essential for development of an evidence-based approach to assessing how well these programmes are doing in preparing graduates for their professional roles and responsibilities. Such a database would provide opportunities for cross-national comparisons of programmes and assessments of their effectiveness in preparing graduates for various roles. It would assist in examining the success of these programmes as well as the attrition they experience, the costs and benefits to society and the healthcare systems that depend on these graduates. It also would provide an opportunity for assessing the perspectives of stakeholders, including the graduates themselves.
2. *Infuse current nursing doctoral curricula with recommendations already available about doctoral education.* As discussed previously, a number of core competencies have already been identified as essential for today's doctoral graduate. These include the types of knowledge and skills for doctorally prepared individuals to function effectively in a variety of organizational contexts across the spectrum of educational, governmental and corporate settings. The competencies identified by the Re-envisioning the PhD Project are applicable to all disciplines, including nursing.

   An excellent example is found at the Graduate School at the University of Texas. This institution offers a series of cross-disciplinary seminars for students in all disciplines throughout their doctoral programmes around the theme of 'intellectual entrepreneurship.' These interdisciplinary learning experiences teach students how to take risks, seize opportunities, discover knowledge through research questions that have direct relevance to pressing problems people face in their social milieu, use innovative strategies to solve complex problems in diverse social realms, collaborate and assume roles as citizen-scholars. Other topics include social ethics, issues related to technology, and integrity in leadership roles (Cherwitz and Sullivan, 2002). All doctoral students, including those in nursing, would benefit from this kind of learning as they also acquire discipline-specific competencies and methods.

3 *Development of global partnerships in nursing education.* Collaborative efforts among nursing doctoral programmes through the development of partnerships would provide powerful learning opportunities in this rapidly changing environment. Doctoral education is in various stages of development in different countries and learning from each other's successes and failures would be efficient and cost-effective. Some of these partnerships and collaborative models have already begun for curricula and mentoring purposes and these could be replicated and expanded. Their experiences can inform others at earlier stages of development. Little seems to be known about how effective programmes are in preparing graduates for their future roles, particularly in the international community (Carty et al, 2002). Since all social systems are challenged today to provide quality services in an environment of diminishing resources, partnerships can provide a mechanism for dialogue and strategic initiatives to address the needed competencies for doctoral nursing graduates today.

Exhibit: Case study profiles of doctorally prepared nurses

Example 1

After completing a Diploma of Nursing in her own country in 1988 Graduate 1 was employed as a registered nurse in an emergency department and a medical ward for two years and then as a school nurse in a rural area for one year, before applying to undertake a Bachelor of Health Science in Nursing conversion programme in Australia. After graduating with this degree, she enrolled in Master of Nursing by research at the same Australian university. As an overseas nurse she underwent an accreditation process in Australia so that she could practise part time while completing her studies. She found employment as an overseas student assistant in the university's international student office during the next two years. She then returned to her own country and worked for two years as a lecturer in emergency medicine and emergency care skills in a health college. However, her ultimate goal was to obtain a PhD in the field of mental health nursing because of her interest in nurse–patient–family interaction. It was also an expectation in her country that an academic career required doctoral level preparation. She accepted the offer of an Australian university PhD scholarship in 1998 and undertook a naturalistic inquiry of the relationships between family carers of people with a mental illness and community mental health nurses. Her supervisors encouraged her to publish and present at conferences during the candidature, which assisted in obtaining a research position prior to graduating. During the candidature she worked as a part-time tutor of nursing students in the faculty and also as a workshop facilitator in problem-based learning within a dedicated problem-based learning centre at the university. Developing these skills provided opportunities to facilitate workshops in this approach to learning in her home county and in Australia, and to assist student learning through translation support. She was awarded the degree in 2002.

Having observed the breadth of research potential in Australia, available only through a long period of apprenticeship in her own country, she decided to seek permanent residency in Australia and establish herself as a researcher. She has held a full-time research position in a health service-based research unit since 2001 and is a research associate with a linked university. These positions provide broad-ranging opportunities to conduct research in the field of aged care, coordinate and manage multidisciplinary research projects, mentor research students and health staff in research, contribute to health service planning and policy development, and network with health staff, consumers and researchers in this specialty field. While the PhD provided her the necessary knowledge and skills to undertake indepth qualitative research, this position has offered new opportunities for a wide range of research processes and areas of inquiry through mentoring. She received a research award within the first year of taking up this position and has been successful in achieving research grants and publications. The PhD, combined with her research training in this new position, provides her with a possible future in the university sector, in a range of health organizations, government departments or in the field of health policy and planning in the non-government sector. Whatever opportunities present, she will have the necessary background for success.

Example 2

After completing an undergraduate degree in business administration at a university in the USA in 1988, Nurse 2 worked for a large management consulting firm. He assisted organizations in the human services industry to find more efficient ways to design and deliver their services in the challenged economic environment. As organizations were rapidly downsizing, these consultations were intended to increase efficiency without compromising the quality or quantity of services provided. As he worked across these organizations, he became increasingly interested in the pressing human needs these organizations were struggling with and decided that he, too, wanted to be more involved in the direct delivery of meeting these pressing social needs. In 1995, he enrolled in an accelerated baccalaureate nursing programme which recognized his previous university education and his background in the business world. The curriculum provided nursing preparation in 14 months, focusing only on the courses needed for professional nursing practice and not requiring any repetition of previous coursework he had completed.

Upon graduation he worked in a critical care unit for two years in a large academic health centre. Experiencing the major issues that nurses faced in hospital-based practice, he yearned to apply his previous management skills in ways that might redesign nursing practice and delivery services of better quality and efficiency. He decided to enroll in a post-baccalaureate doctoral programme in nursing that emphasized nursing systems administration and research. He completed the programme in 2000 and worked for a large healthcare consulting firm that focused on quality improvement and evidence-based practice in the delivery of healthcare services. In 2003, he left that organization and developed his own consulting firm.

References

American Association of Colleges of Nursing (AACN) (2002). *Nursing faculty shortage fact sheet.* Online. Available at: http://www.aacn.nche.edu/Media/Backgrounders/facultyshortage.htm (accessed on 06.03.2003).

AACN Task Force on Future Faculty (2003). *AACN White paper: Faculty shortages in baccalaureate and graduate nursing programs: Scope of the problem and strategies for expanding the supply.* Available at: http://www.aacn.nche.edu/Publications/WhitePapers/FacultyShortages.htm. (accessed on 25.05.2003).

AACN (2002). *Enrollment and graduations in baccalaureate and graduate programs in nursing, 2001–2002.* Washington, DC: AACN.

Atwell, R. H. (1996). Doctoral education must match the nation's needs and the realities of the marketplace. *The Chronicle of Higher Education*, **43**(14), B4–B6.

Australia Education and Training. Employment (2002). *Higher education students time series tables 2001 graduate destination survey.* Australia: Australia Education and Training.

Bazely, P. (2003). Defining 'early career' in research. *Higher Education*, **45**, 257–279.

Berlin, L. E., and Sechrist, K. R. (2002). The shortage of doctorally prepared nursing faculty: A dire situation. *Nursing Outlook*, **50**(2), 50–56.

Berlin, L. E., Stennett, J. and Bednash, G. D. (2003). *Enrollment and graduations in baccalaureate and graduate programs in nursing*. Washington, DC: AACN.

Brennan, M. B. (1997). PhDs face new job market realities. *Chemical & Engineering News*, **75**(11), 47–53.

Carty, R., O'Grady, E. T., Wichaikhum, O. and Bull, J. (2002). Opportunities in preparing global leaders in nursing. *Journal of Professional Nursing*, **18**(2), 70–77.

Cheng, L. T. W. and Davidson, W. N. (2001). The characteristics of job applicants for finance faculty positions: 1986 to 1992. *Financial Practice & Education*, **59**(2), 19–29.

Cherwitz, R. A. and Sullivan, C. A. (2002). Intellectual entrepreneurship: A vision for graduate education. *Change: The Magazine of Higher Learning*, **34**(6), 23–27.

Committee on Dimensions, Causes, and Implications of Recent Trends in the Careers of Life Scientists (1998). *Trends in the Early Careers of Life Scientists*. National Research Council, Washington, DC: National Academy Press.

Delamont, S., Atkinson, P. and Parry, O. (2000). *The Doctoral Experience: Success and Failure in Graduate School*. London: Falmer Press.

Deneef, A. L. (2000). Discussion group notes from: *The purpose of the PhD as preparation for employment: PMLA*. Publication of the Modern Languages Association of America. Available at http://www. . ./pqdlink?Ver=1&Exp=04-15-2003&FMT=ABS&DID=00000006870854&REQ=1&CERT (accessed on 17.03.2003).

Fogg, P. (2003). Family time: Why some women quit their coveted tenure-track jobs. *The Chronicle of Higher Education*, **49**(40), A10–A12.

Gaff, J. G. (2002). Preparing future faculty and doctoral education. *Change: The Magazine of Higher Learning*, **34**(6), 63–66.

Golde, C. M., and Fiske, P. (2000). *Graduate school and the job market of the 1990s: A survey of young geoscientists*. Available at: http://www.agu.org/eos_elec/97117e:html (accessed on 17.03.2003).

Hertel, J., West, T. F., Buckley, W. E. and Denegar, C.R. (2001). Educational history, employment characteristics, and desired competencies of doctoral-educated athletic trainers. *Journal of Athletic Training*, **36**(1), 49–57.

Hoffer, T., Dugoni, B., Sanderson, A., Sederstrom, S., Ghadialy, R. and Rocque, P. (2001). *Doctorate Recipients from United States Universities: Summary Report 2000*. Chicago, IL: National Opinion Research Center.

Horn, M. (1999). 'A practical turn in PhDs. *U.S. News & World Report*, **126**(12): 114.

Hult, D. F. (2000). Playing by the numbers: A different perspective on the job market. *PMLA, Publication of the Modern Languages Association of America*, **115**(5): 1269–1272.

INDEN. (2003). Directory of International Doctoral Programs. International Network for Doctoral Education in Nursing. Available at: http://www.umich.edu/~inden/programs/ (accessed on 01.06.2003).

Ketefian, S. and Redman, R. W. (2001). Global perspectives on graduate nursing education: Opportunities and challenges. In: N. Chaska (ed.). *The nursing profession: Tomorrow and beyond*. Thousand Oaks, CA: Sage Publications.

Ketefian, S., Neves, E. P., and Gutierrez, M. G. (2001). Nursing doctoral education in the Americas. *Online Journal of Issues in Nursing*. Available at: http://www.nursingworld.org/ojin/topic12/tpc12_8.htm (accessed on 19.03.2003).

LaPidus, J. B. (1996). Scholarship and the future of graduate education in science and engineering. Paper presented at the Radcliffe/CPST Conference Science careers, gender equity, and the changing economy. College Park, MD, 1996.

LaPidus, J. B. (1997). Why pursuing a PhD is a risky business. *The Chronicle of Higher Education,* **44**(12), A60. Available at: http://www.grad.washington.edu/envision/project_resources. . ./biblio_over_production.htm (accessed on 17.03.2003).

Lieberman, L. W. (1997). Psychologists as psychotherapists. *The American Psychologist,* **52**(2), 181–183.

Lovitts, B. E. (2001). *Leaving the ivory tower: The causes and consequences of departure from doctoral study*. London: Rowman & Littlefield.

McKenna, H. and Cutcliffe, J. (2001). Nursing doctoral education in the United Kingdom and Ireland. *Online Journal of Issues in Nursing*. Available at: http://www.nursingworld.org/ojin/topic12/tpc12_9.htm. (accessed on 19.03.2003).

McGinn, D. (2000). A PhD hits the road. *Newsweek*, **136**(20), 70–72.

Magner, D. K. (1998). Job market blues. *The Chronicle of Higher Education,* **40**(34), A17–A19.

Malveaux, J. (1995). Education pipeline or merry-go-round. *Black Issues in Higher Education,* **12**(16), 40.

Mangematin, V., Mandran, N. and Crozet, A. (2000). The careers of social science doctoral graduates in France. *European Journal of Education,* **35**(1), 111–125.

Moyer, A. and Salovey, P. (1999). Challenges facing female doctoral students and recent graduates. *Psychology of Women Quarterly,* **23**(3), 607– 631.

Nyquist, J. D. (2002). The PhD: A tapestry of change for the 21st Century. *Change: The Magazine of Higher Learning,* **34**(6), 12–20.

Nyquist, J. D. and Woodford, B. J. (2002). *Re-envisioning the PhD: What Concerns Do We Have?* Available at: http://www.grad.washington.edu/envision/project_resources/ (accessed on 15.03.2003).

Phillips, H. (1998). Investigating the alternatives. *Nature,* **393**(4), 493–495.

Randolph, D. L. (1990). Changing the non-psychology doctorate in counsellor education: A proposal. *Counsellor Education and Supervision*, **30**(2), 135–148.

Redman, R. W. and Ketefian, S. (1997). The changing face of graduate education. In: J. McCloskey and H. Grace (eds). *Current Issues in Nursing*. 5th edn. St Louis, MO: Mosby.

Siegfried, J. J., and Stock, W. A. (1999). The labour market for new PhD economists. *Journal of Economic Perspectives,* **13**(3), 115–135.

Smallwood, S. (2001). Psychology PhDs pass on academe: Star graduates turn down faculty jobs, finding better pay and less stress in industry. *The Chronicle of Higher Education,* **47**(118), A10–A13.

Smith, J., McKnight, A. and Naylor, R. (2000). Graduate employability: Policy and performance in higher education in the UK. *Economic Journal,* **110**(1464), F382–F412.

Taylor, R. D., and Hardy, C. A. (1996). Careers in psychology at the associate's, bachelor's, master's and doctoral levels. *Psychological Reports,* **79**(3), 960–963.

Williams, B. S. (1996). Opportunities in nursing. *The Black Collegian,* **26**(2), 48–52.

Wolff, M. F. (1995). US science and engineering graduates: How many and how are they employed? *Research, Technology, Management,* **38**(5), 6–8.

Xiao, H. (2000). Doctoral graduates: whither away? *Chinese Education & Society,* **33**(5), 81–87.

Yin, J. (1998). Placement report: Political science PhDs and ABDs on the job market in 1997. *PS: Political Science & Politics,* **31**(4), 818–828.

Zimpfer, D. G. and DeTrude, J. C. (1990). Follow-up of doctoral graduates in counseling. *Journal of Counseling & Development,* **69**, 51–56.

Chapter 6

Faculty shortages in doctoral nursing programmes

Shaké Ketefian, Joanne Olson and Hugh P. McKenna

The most important resource for doctoral nursing education programmes is the faculty (Wood and Ross-Kerr, 2003), if the stated purpose of doctoral education for preparing scholars and scientists who will develop disciplinary knowledge is to be fulfilled. Recruitment and retention of qualified faculty members creates a major challenge for leaders in developing and sustaining quality doctoral programmes. As nursing and nursing education advance worldwide, there is an increasing need for doctoral nursing programmes. Likewise, there is a growing need for qualified faculty to offer mentorship and guidance to graduate students studying in doctoral programmes. This chapter focuses on the worldwide faculty shortage in doctoral programmes, and possible reasons for such shortages. We will give examples of the prevalence of this faculty shortage in several countries and discuss the relationship between the nursing shortage in general and the faculty shortage in doctoral programmes. The challenges of faculty recruitment, retention and return will be discussed as well as the effects of faculty shortage on recruitment and retention of doctoral students. Finally, we will discuss creative solutions to the problems presented and give examples of strategies already in use to address faculty shortages in doctoral programmes.

Prevalence of faculty shortages in doctoral programmes

In Canada, the need for doctorally prepared faculty continues to increase for a variety of reasons. First and foremost, over the past 12 years, the number of Canadian doctoral nursing programmes has increased from one in 1991 to 11 in 2003. In addition, the earlier programmes that began with limited numbers of doctoral students are now expanding. As the number of doctoral programmes increases and the student numbers in each programme increase, there is a corresponding need for qualified faculty. At the same time, Canadian nursing continues to move towards baccalaureate level entry for practice. Schools of nursing across the country are therefore seeking doctorally prepared faculty to offer leadership in a growing number of undergraduate programmes. Also, governments across Canada are increasing the numbers of seats allotted to nursing programmes to prepare an appropriate number of nurses for the changing Canadian population of the future. As a result of all of these factors, Canadian educational institutions face severe shortages of adequately prepared faculty for the growing number of undergraduate and graduate programmes (Association of Universities and Colleges of Canada (AUCC), 2002). While the number of nursing education seats filled across Canada has increased by approximately 40% between 1998/99 and 2000/01 (O'Brien-Pallas et al, 2002), and is expected to continue increasing, the number of faculty members is predicted to decrease. This decrease is due largely to the fact that 49.6% of university professors and 37.7% of college instructors will retire by 2010 (Association of Colleges of Applied Arts and Technology, 2001).

While geographically close, the dynamics of faculty shortages in the USA are quite different from those seen in Canada. Some basic statistics will help to put the picture in perspective: despite concerted efforts by the profession and governmental agencies to have at least 1–2% of nurses educated at the doctoral level, as of the year 2000, only 0.6% of all nurses in the USA held a doctorate. Only 82% of these are employed in nursing; 66% of those not employed are 55 years or older, suggesting a relatively early retirement age. The average age of faculty was 52.6 years; the average age when the doctoral degree was received was 43.9 years; and 20.8 years had elapsed between receipt of basic nursing education and the doctoral degree (Geolot, 2003).

These figures reflect a longstanding tradition that has built around graduate nursing education; it is only recently that we have come to realize its negative ramifications. In the USA, for example, the average age of assistant professors (with doctoral preparation) is 50.4 years (Berlin et al, 2002). Due to late entry into doctoral study and late graduation, individuals with doctorates assume beginning faculty positions in their mid-forties, at a time when other faculty are attaining seniority. This leaves them 15–20 years during which they have to develop into expert teachers, obtain significant external funding for their programmatic research in an area of nursing science, publish their findings and have serious impact on practice. They also have to provide leadership within the profession at the national and international levels and become acknowledged as experts (Hinshaw and Ketefian, 2001). Clearly, the short time available to these individuals is insufficient to build the kind of scholarly academic careers expected of senior university faculty, and creates a high degree of pressure and stress in these individuals that is counterproductive.

In the next 5–10 years large numbers of nursing faculty are expected to retire. Some institutions are developing plans to hire a certain number of new graduates each year to groom them to fill the expected vacancies. At the same time, many states across the USA are in financial crises and are reducing their budgets, including that of the universities they support. Thus the plans some institutions have made are not being realized due to retrenchment as a result of budget constraints.

Relationship between nursing shortage and faculty shortage

Some of the increased need for doctorally prepared faculty in North American countries relates directly to the increased need for nurses in general. These countries will need increased numbers of nurses to provide care required for an increasing proportion of elderly people in the population. Some of the increased need for nurses also relates to the decline in the number of registered nursing graduates each year. In Canada, for example, the numbers have decreased from approximately 8000 graduates per year in the early 1990s to 4000 graduates in the year 2000 (Ryten, 2002). The Ryten Report suggests that approximately 12,000 nursing graduates are required per year to sustain the nursing profession. While approximately 12,000 registered nursing students enroll in Canadian nursing programmes each year (O'Brien-Pallas et al, 2002), there is approximately a 30–50% attrition rate (Registered Nurses Association of Ontario, 2002). The shortages of nurses in general led to governments increasing the number of seats in educational institutions preparing nurses and this in turn leads to a need for increased numbers of qualified faculty members.

Nursing shortages are reported in various countries around the world, with varying causes. For example, Thailand is undergoing healthcare reform, following adoption of a new constitution. The philosophy and concept of universal health coverage has been adopted, which requires that 10,000 health centres around the country be staffed by professional nurses, and many do not have qualified nurses yet. Finland reports a nursing shortage, which is expected to get worse as the population ages, while the Netherlands and Sweden report shortages in specialized areas of practice rather than across the board.

The USA has been experiencing a severe shortage of nurses for a number of years. This situation, while serious, has been a cyclical occurrence since the late 1940s and in different eras, different explanations have been offered by economists, nurses and policy makers. Some of these shortages have occurred during economic downturns, but others have not. During economic hard times, schools of nursing have seen an increase in the number of graduate students enrolled at the master's and doctoral levels. Currently, while the nursing shortage continues, there has been no appreciable decrease in applications and enrolment into doctoral programmes. This is not an unreasonable picture, when one remembers that, typically, 15–20 years elapse before most individuals begin doctoral study following graduation from their basic nursing education programmes, so that the pool of applicants for these programmes is not newly graduating individuals, but rather, those who have been in practice for some time.

In Europe, shortage of nurses has been developing since the 1980s. The main reason for this was the view of some conservative governments that there were too many nurses and that unqualified nursing aides could undertake much of nursing work. Furthermore, the number of other non-nursing university degree programmes that were open to young women increased, making it easier for them to gain a place in medical school or fields such as engineering, mathematics and architecture. This, alongside a trend towards smaller family size, meant that the recruitment pool for nursing schools was shrinking.

Across Europe, the response to the shortage of nurses has been threefold: increase in number of nursing students and nursing schools, increase in recruitment from overseas (mostly from the Philippines) and introduction of initiatives to recruit, retain and encourage nurses to return to the profession. The first of these initiatives has had great implications for university schools of nursing.

Unlike the USA, Australia and Canada, nursing within Europe has only recently entered the university sector. In the UK, for instance, there were only ten university-based schools of nursing in the early 1990s. Due to changes in governmental policies and mandates, today there are 72, each requiring well-qualified faculty. Other European countries have experienced similar, though more modest increases.

Many of the faculty who were recruited came from hospital-based schools of nursing which were not affiliated with universities. Hence, they were not qualified at the doctoral level and in some cases did not even possess a baccalaureate degree. They tended to be experienced in teaching and in administrating educational programmes and soon realized that the route to better pay and promotion within the universities was through research and publication. Therefore, many enrolled in doctoral programmes on a part-time basis while holding down heavy teaching and administration roles. Furthermore, many were, and continue to be, over the age of 50. This age is even higher than that reported for the USA.

In some European countries, the increase in the number of faculty undertaking doctoral studies has been matched by an increase in the number of doctoral students who are not faculty. These individuals tend to be clinically based, over the age of 35, who begin doctoral study because they are disenchanted by clinical nursing and wish to find a job in the burgeoning university schools of nursing. In contrast, some individuals from this group are seeking to obtain a doctorate so that they could obtain a promotion to a clinically based advanced nursing practice role.

As in other countries and regions, there is a shortage of faculty with doctoral degrees in Europe. This has implications for the mentoring of the increased number of doctoral students referred to above. Some faculty have taken early retirement or simply resigned because of stress caused by trying to juggle research, teaching, administration and clinical roles. With improvements in pay and conditions within clinical settings and the drive there for research expertise, many of these have gained employment in hospitals.

The adequacy of faculty numbers and the level of their qualifications vary greatly across countries. Some countries report having a sufficient number of graduate programmes, but at the same time, experience faculty shortages. Most countries desire a doctoral qualification for teaching at the graduate level, but have not achieved this goal. In some cases master's-prepared individuals are teaching at the graduate level due to insufficient number of faculty qualified at the doctoral level. Another 'cost' that is paid but not frequently discussed is the reality that due to insufficient number of qualified faculty, the workload of those with appropriate qualifications is so heavy that it precludes research activity, which seems to be sacrificed to make room for more teaching responsibilities. Additionally, some countries are in the process of educating more individuals at the doctoral level, but upon assuming faculty roles, these new faculty are given limited graduate teaching responsibilities due to their inexperience; they themselves need some years of mentoring before they can mentor graduate students. In the case of other countries, the shortage is that of positions not being available or funded, rather than having a shortage of individuals, who could be recruited and hired were funding to be made available. In these instances individuals with doctoral preparation work in a variety of settings while, in some countries such as Brazil, doctoral graduates work mainly in faculty roles, as there is not sufficient appreciation or understanding in other sectors and markets of the type of contribution such individuals can make.

As the examples from Canada, the USA and Europe illustrate, each country presents its own dynamic reasons and factors that impinge on nurse faculty supply. It needs to be noted that some countries do not report shortages. However, this has to be seen in perspective, and one has to consider who is doing the reporting, and for what purpose. For example, the nurses in the Philippines report a severe shortage of nursing and nursing faculty, yet, the country is a major exporter of nurses. The Philippines was the first country in the world that standardized its educational system by offering all nursing education within four-year colleges and universities. It now produces more qualified nurses than the country can absorb; therefore, it has become a major exporter of nurses to the rest of the world. These nurses travel elsewhere and earn higher wages than they would be able to at home, and send funds to support their families, thus contributing to the national economy in significant ways. In Europe, hospital managers have recruited many Filipino nurses. These nurses can get five times the salary they get in the Philippines. This has had the effect of Filipino doctors training to be nurses so that they can get a job overseas.

The question that still needs to be answered is Does the Philippines have a nursing shortage? Those assessing the health care system in that country would give a resounding yes answer. Those taking an economic view of the picture would say that the country cannot employ these nurses, nor would most nurses prefer to work at the low salaries they would receive in their home country, and that exporting them makes sense for the country when considering the overall economic health of the country. In some other countries such as Brazil, the number of nursing personnel has been historically insufficient, a situation that has led to the creation of different type of personnel to meet the needs of the population.

Faculty recruitment issues

Throughout history, Canadian university nursing administrators have experienced difficulty in securing faculty qualified to teach in university programmes. This situation first occurred during the establishment of baccalaureate programmes within universities and is now encountered by administrators attempting to staff developing doctoral programmes with qualified faculty (Wood and Ross-Kerr, 2003). Wood and Ross-Kerr believe that only part of the situation results from a supply and demand issue. They challenge administrators to be perceptive and aggressive in recognizing the skills and potential of faculty members, so that those who show promise can be encouraged and supported in their continual career development.

Other issues that challenge nursing administrators when staffing doctoral programmes include the fact that there are more attractive payment opportunities in the public and private sectors than those offered to new academic faculty. For example, there may be limited start-up funding for research programme development as well as decreasing numbers of faculty support services. Benefits for new as well as continuing faculty members seem to be decreasing as fiscal challenges face universities in general. Unlike Europe, some of the longstanding attractive benefits such as staff and family tuition fee remission in North American universities are being eliminated from benefit packages.

Recruitment efforts have been largely unsuccessful in filling the current and predicted faculty vacancies as well as the new faculty positions being added to promote growth of nursing programmes. As a result, some university schools of nursing have sought qualified academics from outside of Canada. Such recruitment efforts bring both benefits and challenges. The benefits include the blending of new, fresh ideas from other parts of the world with more traditional North American ways of managing nursing education and research. However, there are many challenges to consider when recruiting faculty from other parts of the world. First, the learning curve for faculty coming from other countries is steep and the adjustments required of the faculty member and any associated family members are challenging. The time it takes such faculty members to become fully contributing is often longer than that required for new faculty from the same country. In addition, there is a concern that such recruitment efforts may 'poach' excellent faculty from other parts of the world where their leadership skills are also desperately required. Finally, the provincial/state RN licensing body requirements are often difficult for academics from other counties to meet. Many have been more involved in research than in direct clinical nursing while they studied in their own doctoral programmes. Therefore, intense study time and additional clinical practice are sometimes required to gain current clinical knowledge. Some new faculty members from other countries speak two or three languages but English is usually not their first language. However, North American licensing exams are written in English, so new faculty members are required to write their examinations in a language other than their own. This can be a major challenge. Others are quite challenged by the exam format. Some are more comfortable with essay-type exams than they are with the multiple-choice type exams that are standard in the North American systems for registration. While recruitment of faculty from other countries can be beneficial in the long run, the initial investment is major for both the individual faculty member involved and the host school of nursing.

The pool for nurse faculty: the pipeline problem

For years, when faced with a shortage of any kind, the US response has tended to be to find money as a way of solving the problem. An important concern with regard to faculty shortage has been how to increase the pool from which faculty are drawn, in other words, how to address the 'pipeline' problem. A national initiative is now under way to recruit doctoral students from those who are graduating from their basic programmes, and get them excited and interested in graduate work even while they are early in their undergraduate years. Faculty are now being assigned to mentor highly promising students and incorporate them into their research teams, providing them with stimulating opportunities so they can see the possibilities of nursing research for developing nursing science and improving the health of citizens. This type of early coaching and guiding has yielded a pool of young and energetic applicants to doctoral programmes. This group promises to energize our doctoral student body and create a new pool of future academics who will be ready to assume positions in their late twenties or early thirties. Funds are being sought from private foundations as well as the National Institute of Nursing Research to support such individuals during their doctoral work (Hinshaw and Ketefian, 2001).

This path is not without its problems. It proposes a break from the old tradition, to establish a new tradition in nursing. In some institutions we see a situation that while one group of faculty are working towards recruiting strong undergraduates towards early doctoral work, another group of faculty, mainly those who supervise students' clinical work, are counselling these same students that they should first graduate and work for a while to gain experience. It is therefore critical that a faculty group discuss these issues and come to philosophical agreements about the approach being taken so that as a group, they speak with one voice.

The idea of having some experience in nursing at the start of one's career is one that has merit. In a practice discipline, the problems that arise in practice are a crucial starting place for generating research questions for investigation that will then have real impact in improving the health and quality of life of citizens. The challenge is how experience is interpreted and operationalized, and how much experience is deemed sufficient. Some institutions who admit these young graduates to their doctoral programmes are working out arrangements with health facilities to employ these students as part-time interns, with pay, and are pairing them with experienced and highly professionalized staff nurses who will serve as excellent role models for these novices (Hinshaw and Ketefian, 2001). This type of mentored experience can continue for a year or two until the new graduate has a solid grounding in an area of practice, and has sufficient familiarity with the context of care. When she or he is ready to begin research, there is sufficient appreciation of practice issues and problems so that the individual can draw on these in formulating research questions. Other institutions are developing other solutions to these problems. We are in an exploratory mode as far as this issue is concerned; while the solutions and answers are not firmed up, the awareness of the problem is present and being addressed actively.

Within the USA there have been dramatic increases in the number of doctoral programmes over the past 20 years. However, neither the number of overall enrolled doctoral students, nor the total number of graduates each year has shown appreciable increases. For example, in 1997 there were 68 doctoral programmes, with 433 graduates nationally, while in 2002, with 81 doctoral programmes reporting, there were 457 graduates overall (Berlin, 2003). This picture suggests that there is inefficiency in the system, with increasing numbers of doctoral programmes recruiting faculty, to in effect educate the same number of overall students system-wide. When one considers the anecdotal reports regarding the increased number of international students studying within the USA for their doctoral degrees (exact numbers are not available), the picture becomes even murkier. Institutions are recruiting faculty from two distinct pools at present: one is the pool of new doctoral graduates; and the second is from faculty members who are already functioning in faculty roles in other institutions and are of senior rank. In an effort to attract from the second pool especially, many institutions are offering attractive packages, such as promotion/tenure, prestigious endowed professorships, start-up funds for research, lab space and facilities for research, better pay, and the like. However, none of these strategies helps increase the available pool of faculty.

Another interesting phenomenon that has exacerbated the insufficiency of the traditional pool of new doctoral graduates available for recruitment is an increase in the percentage of doctoral graduates indicating plans for employment outside education. For the 1980–1984 graduates, 15.5% expected to be employed outside education, while for the 1995–1999 graduates, 26.9% expected to be employed outside education (National Opinion Research Center, 2001).

Unlike the USA or Canada, movement of faculty across Europe is not common. This is mainly due to language barriers and differences in legislation and regulations. However, within countries it is common for university schools of nursing to poach faculty from other schools. Possession of a doctorate and a good publication and grant award record make faculty attractive to other universities. Incentives are often offered in terms of tenure, pay, research and secretarial support. Furthermore, it is often easier to get promotion in another university than in one's own and this sometimes stimulates movement of faculty from one school of nursing to another.

There is much that can be done to encourage recruitment of students into doctoral programmes and from there into faculty positions. However, many of these lessons have yet to be learned. For instance, on graduating, high-performing students in many European schools of nursing are not encouraged to commence doctoral studies. Rather, they are told to gain three years' experience as a nurse in a clinical setting. For many reasons including marriage and career advancement, most of these students do not return to the university to study or to work. As in the USA and Canada, some nursing schools are beginning to encourage these graduates to stay on and undertake a doctorate part-time while building up their clinical experience.

Faculty retention issues

Retaining good faculty members is the next challenge facing university nursing administrators once successful recruitment has occurred. With increased competition for qualified faculty, excellent faculty members are in a 'recruitable' position, especially after some academic experience in their first appointment. To retain excellent faculty, schools of nursing need to invest heavily in faculty development and continuing professional development programme opportunities. In addition, efforts to mentor, coach, and support developing academics is crucial. More seasoned faculty members need to be encouraged to see faculty development as part of their roles and rewarded for their efforts in this area.

Retention of good faculty members is especially important as increasing demands for productivity are being placed on new academics. The requirements to obtain research funding and to publish in peer-reviewed journals continue as always, but the competition surrounding these marks of success has become increasingly severe. As well, other scholarly pursuits, a good teaching record, and useful community service are expected of new faculty members. Added to these expectations are the increased requirements for an active clinical practice that relates to one's research programme and the need to work collaboratively within interdisciplinary research groups. Mentorship is desperately needed but often lacking for the development of new faculty members for all of these roles. But, in addition to learning these new roles, faculty members need the guidance of more seasoned academics so that they learn to live satisfying, balanced lives in the midst of such heavy career demands.

Sometimes, because of inadequate 'manpower' or lack of succession planning, new academics are catapulted into leadership roles almost the moment they complete doctoral education. In addition to placing them in these roles before they may be ready, this action jeopardizes their potential to develop a strong research career during the initial years in academia. Neither the nursing profession nor the individual's career benefits from such hasty movement into leadership positions. This situation is a special problem in countries where the number of individuals with doctoral preparation is small; upon return to their country from overseas study, many face a 'reality shock' and are expected to carry heavy teaching and advisement loads, thus delaying the initiation of research and scholarly activities by many years, and engendering a degree of alienation and frustration that is counterproductive.

Returning faculty

In parts of Europe there is a policy of encouraging faculty who have resigned or retired to return to work. Many of these individuals had left jobs in education because they wanted to raise a young family or because they had moved elsewhere because their partner had changed jobs. As alluded to above, others had taken early retirement due to work pressures. The stimulus for encouraging their return is not just the shortages of faculty but the experience and knowledge that these people bring back with them. Young faculty need mentoring from such experienced colleagues and because of their experience they can often take on administration roles, which free up younger faculty to focus on research and completing their doctorates.

Universities need to put together a portfolio of incentives to attract faculty back to work. These include child care, good pay, flexible working such as job sharing, family-friendly hours and duties and promotion criteria that take into account part-time faculty.

In the USA, nurses working in clinical settings can earn higher salaries than nursing faculty. Currently, this is not the case in Europe; however, because of the shortage of clinically-based nurses, some European governments are introducing improved terms and conditions for practising nurses. It is predicted that this will cause major recruitment and retention problems for universities. For instance, in the UK, there are 6900 full-time university-based nursing faculty; to lose even a small proportion of these to clinical roles could threaten the viability of some educational and research programmes.

Effects of faculty shortage on students in doctoral programmes

The goal of doctoral study is to prepare scholars and scientists who will develop knowledge for their discipline and who will be leaders. Research training occurs best using an apprenticeship model. Students in such an education programme are expected to be involved in their faculty supervisor's research programme. The research programme provides the context for the student's socialization into research and scholarship (Wood and Ross-Kerr, 2003). Shortages of faculty prepared to offer leadership in doctoral programmes directly translate into a limited number of research programmes to which graduate students can connect. Furthermore, with few faculty and a limited number of research programmes in many countries, faculty members are increasingly required to take on more student supervision than may be academically sound. With increased numbers of doctoral students per faculty member, there could be decreased time for individual student attention and direction, and increased time to completion of the doctoral degree as a result, and in some cases, compromise quality.

Creative solutions to the problem of faculty shortage

Several recommendations are proposed below in an effort to address the faculty shortage issues. Different solutions are likely to be appropriate for different settings and situations. Further, it should be noted that each suggested approach may give rise to new problems that need to be recognized and addressed.

- Recruit faculty worldwide – some countries have more doctorally prepared nurses than needed (limited number of positions in small number of universities).
- Seek a work–life balance whereby faculty are not overwhelmed between their home life and pressures for research, teaching, administration and clinical work.
- Introduce family-friendly working hours and conditions to recruit, retain or encourage faculty to return to work.
- Use adjunct faculty appointments to engage doctorally prepared people from the public and private sectors in co-supervision of doctoral students or for serving on doctoral supervisory committees.
- Develop creative educational programming especially for doctoral programmes but also in terms of moving nurses more quickly from basic nursing programmes to completion of doctoral programmes.
- Convince governments to collaborate to fund nursing scholarships and bursaries equivalent to 50% or more of tuition for nurses studying in master's and doctoral programmes (Registered Nurses Association of Ontario, 2002).
- Keep national inventories of tenure track positions available across countries.
- Improve access to educational programmes in areas that do not have ready access to universities – governments and university nursing programmes can collaborate to maximize technology (i.e. distance education) and in-person opportunities for nurses in remote and rural settings (Registered Nurses Association of Ontario, 2002).
- Promote academics in nursing as a career path (Registered Nurses Association of Ontario, 2002).
- Promote partnership posts with clinical settings. This increases the credibility of the faculty member to students, allows access to research subjects in clinical settings and forges strong links between health facilities and universities.
- Investigate and promote non-traditional approaches to graduate education with regard to alternative admission requirements and flexible delivery modes for instruction (Registered Nurses Association of Ontario, 2002).

References

Association of Colleges of Applied Arts and Technology (2001). *The 2001 environmental scan for the Association of Colleges of Applied Arts and Technology of Ontario.* Toronto.

Association of Universities and Colleges of Canada (2002). *Trends in higher education: Summary of findings.* Available at: http://www.aucc.ca/en/publications/publications index.html (accessed on 10.11.2003).

Berlin, L. E. (2003). Future availability of doctorally prepared nursing faculty. Paper presented at the AACN Doctoral Conference, Sanibel Island, Florida, 2003.

Berlin, L. E., Stennett, J. and Bednash, G. D. (2002). *2001–2002 salaries of instructional and administrative faculty in baccalaureate and graduate programs in nursing.* Washington, D.C.

Geolot, D. H. (2003). Doctoral education in nursing. Paper presented at the AACN Doctoral Education Conference, Sanibel Island, Florida, 2003.

Hinshaw, A. S. and Ketefian, S. (2001). Nurse scientist preparation: Fast track for academic nursing. In: *Envisioning doctoral education for the future.* Washington, D.C.: American Association of Colleges of Nursing, pp. 63–75.

National Opinion Research Center (2001). Survey of earned doctorates. Unpublished special reports generated for the American Association of Colleges of Nursing.

O'Brien-Pallas, L., Meyer, R., Alksnis, C. et al. (2002). *Nursing education data – Evaluation of strategy 7 of the Nursing Strategy for Canada.* Report submitted to Health Canada. Toronto: Nursing Effectiveness, Utilization and Outcomes Research Unit, University of Toronto.

Registered Nurses Association of Ontario (2002). *Nursing education think tank 2002 final report.* Toronto.

Ryten, E. (2002). *Planning for the future: Nursing human resource projections.* Ottawa, Canada: Canadian Nurses Association.

Wood, M. J. and Ross-Kerr, J. C. (2003). The growth of graduate education in nursing in Canada. In: J. C. Ross-Kerr and M. J. Wood (eds). *Canadian nursing: Issues and perspectives.* Toronto: Mosby, pp. 466–488.

Chapter 7

The doctoral process: from idea to award

John R. Cutcliffe, Leana Uys and Eun-Ok Lee

Aspirant doctoral students may find comfort in, as the title of this chapter indicates, the description and explanation of 'the' doctoral process. Clearly marked pathways, which arguably suggest a degree of certainty, perhaps help students to feel more secure (Cutcliffe and Goward, 2000). However, the authors of this chapter purport that there is no one, singular doctoral process. The international 'flavour' of the authors and their resultant particularized experiences are testimony to this. Consequently, it would be remiss of the authors if they were to describe 'the' singular process of undertaking a doctorate. Such parochial conceptualizations are perhaps analogous to positing a singular 'research process' or a singular process for nurse preparation and registration.

It would be particularly inappropriate of the authors to describe 'the' singular process for undertaking a doctorate also because the pattern of doctoral education differs somewhat in a number of countries. Fundamental differences exist between those doctoral programmes where students begin their studies with coursework, of varying lengths, one to two or more years,[1] and those programmes where students undertake a doctorate by thesis or dissertation. The steps within a taught doctorate are viewed as preparation for students in undertaking their dissertation research. Yet, it is useful to remember that students who have experienced extensive coursework, have had research experiences with faculty, and have typically moved through their programme with a cohort of students have a different level of support system and resources to draw from than those who have not.

Consequently, what follows in this chapter might be best regarded as a collection of (hopefully) helpful suggestions, based on the authors' experiences of undertaking, completing, supervising and examining doctorate-level education. It would be equally remiss of the authors if they were to assume that their experiences could be generalized to every doctoral candidate. Therefore, the reader may be served best by this chapter by 'trying on' some of the suggestions to see, to paraphrase Barney Glaser (2001), if they have 'fit and grab'. At the very least, the authors believe that, given their international and disparate experiences, there should be something in this chapter that resonates or has meaning for (aspirant) doctoral candidates from around the world.

It is also important to note that while 'the' doctoral process is necessarily described as a linear, sequential process, this is only a description and the experience of undertaking a doctorate may not follow such a linear pattern. There are, for example, many aspects of 'the' doctoral process that are more cyclic in nature (e.g. the writing of the dissertation is not necessarily an activity that occurs *ex post facto*, but should be an ongoing activity). This chapter, accordingly, should be read with this in mind.

Identifying the dissertation topic

On first consideration, identifying the dissertation topic may appear straightforward but the authors would point out that this might not always be the case. Some of the difficulty surrounding this process may be grounded in the different methods of achieving a doctoral degree and the variation in international experiences.[2] For example, the traditional pathway to gaining a doctoral degree in many countries was to undertake a Doctor of Philosophy (PhD) that culminated in the production of a sizeable thesis, usually upwards of 100,000 words (McKenna et al, 2000). In such instances, it was often necessary to identify a topic for research, prepare a proposal (upon which the decision to register or reject the student was made) even before one registered for a doctorate. While contemporary models of doctoral preparation for nurses in many countries tend not to reflect this model and more often follow the taught doctorate model (culminating in a shorter study and smaller thesis), it might be advisable to have a good idea of an area of research before trying to register for a doctoral programme.

However, those aspirant doctoral candidates who undertake coursework within their doctorate (a taught doctorate[3]) are unlikely to be required to identify a dissertation topic prior to admission to the programme. Some would even argue that it would be disadvantageous to do so. In these settings coursework and didactic study occupy an important role in doctoral study. The courses that are taught have different functions. For example, core courses provide foundational knowledge and understanding, such as nursing theory, philosophy of science, development of models which are mental representations of research ideas students bring. Another group of courses consist of research methods, designs and analytic techniques, which students are likely to use in their dissertations. Yet another set of courses consist of advanced nursing science focusing on research in a particular area of nursing knowledge, while another group has courses carefully selected from other disciplines, as they shed light on the student's research problem. Consequently, identifying the topic for study in one's dissertation may well be considerably influenced by participation in these courses. Similarly, according to McKenna and Cutcliffe (2001) an emerging trend is for the supervisor or academic adviser to provide the topic and the research proposal and for the aspirant doctoral student to apply through a competitive process to undertake the work. For example, in addition to the coursework feature, many doctoral programmes in the USA require that students engage in supervised research experience in an aspect of ongoing faculty research. In these instances, clearly the aspirant candidate would not independently select a dissertation topic. The candidate may select a topic in collaboration with his/her supervisor or academic adviser. However, even in such cases the authors assert that, because his or her dissertation will ultimately 'belong' to the candidate and not the supervisor or academic adviser, the candidate needs to consider the choice of topic in great detail.

The choice is an important one, since not only has the candidate to live with it for the years of doctoral study, but also because it should be the foundation of a further research career. This means that the candidate should choose a topic that is rich enough to keep him or her busy for some time; one that has the potential of attracting funding; one that will open up additional research opportunities in the future after graduation and one that may open future employment opportunities. In order to select the topic of dissertation, information outside the university as well as inside the university should be searched through colloquia, seminars, conferences, newsletters, journal reviews, and the supervisor's ideas. In many cases, there exist national funding organizations such as National Institutes of Health in the USA, Canadian Institutes of Health Research, (Medical Research Council of South Africa), and scientific funding agencies that outline specific research priorities every five or ten years. In addition to country-specific organizations, there also exist international bodies (e.g. World Health Organization, European Commission) who set specific research agendas. The organizations and bodies inevitably have websites that should be accessed to get information regarding the selection of a topic for study. Further, organized opportunities for reflection and feedback between graduate students and faculty mentors are necessary in each university. While candidates typically find many opportunities to interact and support each other, many departments structure opportunities to facilitate and encourage discussions among graduate students and faculty about important issues related to the research topics and the methodology.

These longer-term implications of the resultant choice of dissertation topic should not be readily dismissed and perhaps such considerations are illustrative of one potential dilemma facing aspirant candidates. In essence the dilemma facing the student might look something like this; 'Should I select a topic that has contemporary currency or importance[4] or should I select a topic that I believe is equally important to advancing the substantive knowledge base of nursing, that has less contemporary currency or importance right now but may well become politically salient in the future?' It is important to note that many topics that have such contemporary currency (political, practical or theoretical) may have a limited 'shelf-life'. The current 'hot topic' becomes lukewarm; is replaced by the latest 'hot topic' and the funding patterns shift accordingly.[5] Furthermore, there exist many topics that are equally worthwhile of scholarly attention and research yet, hitherto, for many reasons, have remained relatively unexplored, e.g. some mental health related problems. It is also worthy of note that, in some instances, the area of clinical practice of the candidate is so specialized that this suggests an area of research, if not a specific topic. For instance, a nurse working as a clinician in a substance misuse 'outreach' centre or a nurse working as a clinical research assistant in the field of cancer study or chronic diseases would be foolish not to choose a topic closely related to these areas. In other instances it is not so easy.

To summarize this section, the choice should be influenced by the candidate's own interests, clinical specialty and passions. In making this choice, the candidate should be cognizant of the longitudinal nature of research programmes and not limit his or her thinking to the duration of the doctorate. Furthermore, the candidate should be mindful of the contemporary 'hot topics' and the funding opportunities that sometimes accompany such issues while also considering that there remain many substantive issues in nursing which may become 'hot topics' for the future. Doctoral candidates should be aware of the information regarding research topics that is posted on the websites of the various funding organizations and bodies. When the candidate wishes to work on a dissertation topic identified by an academic adviser or potential supervisor, in addition to these considerations, the candidate should consider whether or not his or her interests, passions and personality dovetail the supervisor's.

Writing the proposal

After identification of a dissertation topic, everyone has to continue review of the research articles to clarify the proposal. Although we always talk about 'the proposal' as if there is only one, a candidate might have to write a number of proposals. Again, we recognize that the specific number of proposals will differ depending on the individual practices of the admitting university. Thus, by way of an example, the range of proposals may include, first, an elaborate proposal that one prepares for supervisors and academics to get institutional approval for the dissertation. This is in the first place an academic document, talking to scholars. It needs to convince in terms of scholarly criteria. Secondly, there can be a requirement to write a proposal specifically for a research ethics committee. This is often a shorter proposal and one that enables the candidate to get access to research sites. This is a brief document outlining the research, using more 'accessible' language, often using mainly 'layman's' terms, but focusing strongly on the ethical issues, implications for the service or site, and possible usefulness of the research. It is the practicalities, the operationalization, of the research design that is most important here. Lastly, there is the proposal that is prepared in order to access funding. In this case the proposal needs to address the priorities and criteria of the funding agency in the first instance. Although the substantive content and 'core' of each of these proposals is largely the same, the detail might differ significantly.

Additionally, writing the proposal is perhaps prefaced by a number of processes. Certainly, the candidate will have to engage in a lot of thinking, exploration and reading. A tentative relationship with the doctoral supervisor(s) or academic adviser may need to be established prior to writing the proposal. Depending on the area of study and the potential method,[6] it may be essential to first do a thorough literature review, then identify the research problem, its aim and objectives, and if not already done so, the method, and then commence with the proposal. The proposal should, in essence, make a case for conducting the research (Morse, 1994). It should illustrate the gaps in the current substantive knowledge base and it needs to identify how the proposed research might 'bridge' such gaps (Cutcliffe and Stevenson, 2001). It should provide a logical sequence of steps that illustrate how the candidate intends to carry out the study; where the study will take place; what the intended outcomes of the study are; and how the findings will be disseminated (Tripp-Reimer and Cohen, 1991). It is also important to note that many research studies have an evolutionary or developmental nature.[7] Consequently, the eventual design of the doctoral research study, and sometimes even the research question, may not match that described in the proposal. Such disparity should not be regarded as a limitation, but is perhaps more indicative of the developing methodological and analytical ability of the candidate.

To summarize this section, the writing of the proposal is prefaced by a number of preliminary processes; trying to write a proposal too soon is a waste of time. The proposal should 'make a case' for undertaking the study and should provide the preliminary cadre of the study design. Furthermore, the candidate should write the proposal with the understanding that the design of the study may change as the study progresses, particularly with studies that have an emergent design.

Getting funded

In some countries there are agencies that fund doctoral students by giving them a lump sum (e.g. South Africa), which can be used for any part of the cost of the doctorate. It might be enough to fund the research, depending on the method. Such funding is usually accessed early in the programme, and is not dependent on the proposal being accepted. It might not be enough; thus the authors would urge the doctoral candidate to explore the following options:

- Employers of nurses studying on a part-time basis may be interested in funding the research, especially if it is to be undertaken during the employer's service and if benefits for the organization are visible. Furthermore, there exist some universities that will allow assisted study leave for doctoral candidates.[8]
- If the research supervisor is a funded researcher, it might be possible to obtain 'piggy-back funding'. For example, in South Africa, some grants allow a specific number of Master's, doctoral and postdoctoral student

grants automatically, depending on the rating of the principal investigator. This makes it essential to choose a supervisor carefully, if possible.

- Apply for funding from a provincial, national or international organization working in your area of research. Many organizations have funding for smaller research projects, and such funds could be enough for a doctoral project. Surfing the web is a good way of identifying such potential funders.
- Apply to national research funding agencies. Many countries have such agencies, for example, the National Research Foundation (UK), the Medical Research Council (UK and South Africa), Canadian Institutes of Health Research (Canada) or other funding agencies funded by the governments to support research. For such agencies there are usually recognized channels to apply. Depending on the country of application, some nurses might find it difficult to access such resources, since there is sometimes the perception that only laboratory research and research by medical doctors fall into this category. It might demand advocacy for nursing research by professional and academic organizations to open this resource to nurses. For example, in Korea, the Korean Research Foundation provides funds for doctoral candidates for their dissertations; Korean Nurses Association and Korean Nursing Academies in specific fields of nursing provide some funds for the candidates of the master's programmes.
- Governments or other organisations sometimes put out a call for research tenders or proposals. This is published in specific places, such as government gazettes or on the websites of organizations. Although it is not easy for a beginning researcher to get such funding, it is still a possibility that should be explored.
- The last chapter of this book provides additional pointers on funding.

Obtaining funding is not without its problems. The funding cycle might retard the progress of the candidate – but not as much as a total lack of funding! Funding bodies sometimes demand changes to a proposal that has already been accepted by the university. Or they demand frequent reports that put an additional strain on the time of the candidate. Or they want control over publications. These implications have to be explored before the candidate accepts the funding, since some flexibility might be possible at this early stage. Lastly, it needs to be acknowledged that even without funding, it is still possible to complete a doctorate if the candidate is studying part time. The absence of funding then does not necessarily equate with an inability to complete.

In summary, candidates would be wise to explore a variety of funding options. One refusal for funding should not be regarded as an indication that the study is 'non-fundable'; try again; re-submit; consider alternative funding options. If funding for the complete duration of the study is not available from one funding body then the candidate should seek to 'top up' the funding from alternative sources.

Mode of study

It is often regarded as axiomatic that the choice of research method should be driven by the particular research question and by what is currently known about the phenomenon (Morse and Field, 1994). In addition to those methodological and epistemological considerations, there are a few additional practical issues to be mindful of when choosing a research approach. First, if the candidate has never done qualitative research before, it might be difficult to switch to this approach at doctoral level, or vice versa. Qualitative and quantitative approaches demand different skills and a proven ability in one paradigm (perhaps demonstrated through obtaining a Master's degree) does not necessarily mean that such skills exist in the other paradigm. Such lack of methodological ability might be addressed, to some extent, by undertaking appropriate coursework, and having a supervisor or academic adviser or a committee that is skilled in the approach selected, but the choice needs careful consideration.

Secondly, successfully obtaining funding may also be influenced by the choice of mode of study. While some funding bodies are open-minded about qualitative research, others might discriminate against researchers using this approach. The candidate's choice of mode of study is also likely to be influenced by his or her own philosophical bent. Arguments have been posited that certain disciplines have a greater affinity for (and history of) particular methodological approaches.[9] It is reasonable to posit that similarly, certain individuals will have a greater affinity for particular methodological approaches. There are those people who are most comfortable with positivistic views of the world (i.e. objective truth exists, the world is subject to the laws of science, events outside the mind can be observed, described, explained and predicted, and the researcher can investigate the world from the object–subject standpoint). Such individuals are likely to be drawn to the quantitative paradigm. There are also those people who are most comfortable with naturalistic/interpretivist/constructivist views of the world (i.e. in the social world, reality is constructed, full of shared meanings and inter-subjective realities, constructed and interpreted by those people who inhabit and experience those realities, and the researcher can investigate the world from the standpoint of subject–subject). Thus, such individuals are likely to be drawn to the qualitative paradigm. This is not to suggest that the candidate's own level of comfort with one paradigm or another should be the deciding variable in influencing the mode of study. Nevertheless, it stands to reason that candidates are more likely to be enthusiastic about undertaking a study that complements their own philosophical bent. Given the duration of a doctoral programme, the value of this enthusiasm should not be ignored.

Lastly, the choice might also be influenced by the candidate's career plans. If the candidate plans to work in a large university with a well-developed, multi-paradigmatic research programme, it might be acceptable for the candidate to develop expertise in only one approach, e.g. to be purely a qualitative researcher. However, if the candidate intends to spend his or her academic career in a small university, with a less developed research programme, it is possible that, after graduation, the candidate will have to supervise students in all kinds of approaches. It might therefore serve the candidate well to get experience in both approaches, and not become totally specialized.

In summary, the choice of mode of study is likely to be heavily influenced by the particular research question and by what is currently known about the phenomenon. The candidate's own familiarity and/or greater affinity with a certain research paradigm is likely to have a strong influence on the choice, and the foreseeable academic career pathway of the candidate could also influence the choice of mode of study.

Doing the research

The process of conducting the study is perhaps facilitated by a well-written proposal. The more detailed and well-thought-out the proposal, arguably the study will be easier to implement, even allowing for studies of an emergent design. However, there will undoubtedly be unforeseen problems and difficulties encountered and awareness of such eventualities perhaps makes them easier to manage when they arise. In order to minimize these potential difficulties, the authors would urge the doctoral candidate to consider the following suggestions.

- Try to do what your proposal said you would do.[10]
- It helps to remain focused on your study, while at the same time allowing 'time out.' This is particularly pertinent for part-time students. It is all too easy, in these 'high pressured' days, to be drawn into distraction and become caught up in other work (academic or otherwise). Consequently, candidates will need to learn how to say 'no' and thus retain their focus on their study.
- Stay very close to your data collection. Look at data, in whatever form they take, as they come in – don't just file them for data entry later. Sometimes a candidate can identify problems early enough to correct the problem and while collecting the data can still do something about it. Read interviews immediately, and write down comments or thoughts, before they are forgotten. Time spent during data collection on cleaning and monitoring data is well worth the effort.
- Know your method and stick to it. Similarly, know your research focus and stick to it. It is often tempting to pursue interesting 'side issues' as they emerge, though in so doing, you will be distracted from your study.
- Write as you go. Work step by step, and do not let all the writing to wait until the end. If you write as you go on with the process, you are clearer on how the research is going, and can still adapt or add aspects, or at least

think about what your results are showing. It will also give your supervisor the opportunity to see what you are doing, and allow time for feedback.

- Draw upon all the forms of support that are available – professional and personal. You may need them!
- Maintain your attachments and connections to your academic community. They can be an excellent form of support and can keep you grounded in the 'real world'.[11]
- Lastly, try to publish as you go along. A doctoral study can be conceptualized as producing a series of publications. One does not need to limit oneself to publishing only when the findings are in and the study completed. There may be publishable papers arising from the literature review, the method, the findings and the discussion.

Maintaining motivation

Maintaining motivation is easier when you are researching a phenomenon or issue that you are passionate about, something that is of interest to you; something that has particular meaning for you. Selecting such a topic for study may not always be possible, so additional strategies need to be considered. It may help to conceptualize the 'vision' or as McKenna et al (2000) describe, doctoral study represents the search for the substance; the essential material of the discipline. A doctoral study then has the potential to make a unique and substantive contribution to the discipline and such a vision can be a source of encouragement and motivation in itself. A further method of staying motivated is to recognize that doctoral study is more of a 'long distance' test rather than a 'sprint'. A realistic expectation of such endeavour then is that there will be 'ups and downs' during the process; it is unlikely to be all 'plain sailing'. Candidates are people and people have moods that fluctuate over time, so too will a candidate's motivation. But this is OK, it is usual, it is to be expected. Hence, candidates should not be overly discouraged by periods of low motivation. There may even be merit in 'holidays' from the doctoral study, during which time the candidate should find ways and time to de-stress.

One of the best ways of maintaining your motivation is to have a very clear time schedule and regular appointments with the supervisor or academic adviser. Clear and attainable objectives should be set for each meeting. Even though the candidate does not complete the work, the appointment should still be kept, since it is all too easy to just cancel appointments. The conversation between supervisor and student sometimes identifies barriers to progress, and this allows for motivation to be maintained. Another excellent way to keep motivated is to keep to your planned time schedule. That ensures progress, and it allows you to reach goals and this increases motivation. Once one falls behind, it is difficult to start again. Another way of increasing motivation is to talk about the research to one's colleagues, peers and other students. This can be done informally or formally by scheduling a presentation inside or outside the university. Such presentations give an incentive for progress, and the interest of others by questions and suggestions is motivating for the lagging student.

Being scholarly

It should be noted, with a distinct sense of irony, that defining the process and practice of 'being scholarly' may warrant a doctoral study in itself. Furthermore, there is no 'formula' that one can follow conscientiously in order to become and remain scholarly. Nevertheless, there are a number of practices that are likely to enhance the standard of scholarship and thus help the candidate to 'be scholarly'.

- It is rather obvious, though still worthy of inclusion, that the candidate should read a lot. The foundation of academic study is reading; becoming familiar and conversant with the literature in the substantive area of study. There is also a need to read more widely, candidates are likely to need to read related philosophical, epistemological and methodological literature.
- In addition to acknowledging the value of reading, the true scholar reads literature in a critical way. Candidates need to critique the studies they read (Cutcliffe and Ward, 2003). They need to de-construct the arguments that have been made, consider the methodological rigour, think about why the author has chosen to use these words and not others. They need to contemplate the longitudinal nature of knowledge generation and accumulation. Remembering that knowledge accumulation has a 'horizontal' parameter in addition to the 'vertical' parameter; knowledge accumulation includes having more perspectives from which to know, in addition to knowing more (Sandelowski, 1997).
- A potentially wise, although sometimes difficult, practice is to read one's own thesis and think how it could be criticized by somebody. This is not always easy given the emotional attachment that one develops with one's own work. However, try and ask yourself, if this was a thesis I was examining or reviewing, how would I criticize it, what limitations would I point out, how would I say it could be improved? In this way, one is able to anticipate some of the potential criticisms and limitations that could be identified by an examiner.

A particular section or aspect of doctoral theses which may benefit from additional scholarly attention is the 'Discussion' section. Too often, candidates do not enter into a full, rich, wide discussion of the findings. Scholarly discussions include the implications of the findings in relation to the four areas of practice, education, further research and policy. Furthermore, the discussion should start at the substantive level and evolve to include the formal area. A scholarly discussion, in a nursing thesis, should be able to make some important and illuminative statements about each of these areas. Lastly, thinking in terms of the wider academy of scholars, the scholarship of the candidate's thesis may be enhanced by consideration of how his or her professional work is connected to the needs of other disciplines, society and the global community. Perhaps by working with more than one mentor in different disciplines, the opportunity for interdisciplinary scholarship is enhanced.[12]

Writing-up

A point which must be emphasized, which the authors have already alluded to, is that writing the thesis should not be an activity that occurs *ex post facto*. So, even though this section occurs towards the end of this chapter, in no way is this an indication of when writing-up should occur. Remember the cyclic nature of some doctoral study. For example, if the candidate is using a grounded theory method, the processes of data collection, analysis and writing should occur simultaneously (Glaser and Strauss, 1967). Candidates are often discouraged by the daunting prospect of 'starting to write'. Such a dynamic is more pronounced when the candidate has not undertaken any writing during the bulk of the doctoral study and leaves it for the end. Thus, beginning writing as early as possible can minimize the 'daunting prospect'. Writing a thesis often takes on a rhythm; when this is achieved the writing 'flows', it is fluid and smooth rather than staccato. The authors suggest that in the early stages of writing the candidate should not be overly concerned with producing the perfect piece, or that every sentence is grammatically correct. Just write, as Max van Manen (2002) would say. There are pre-conscious processes occurring during such writing that should not be inhibited by over-attention to grammar. Ideas, insights and conceptualizations will be occurring. The proof-reading and attention to punctuation and grammar can happen later.

As we have stated previously, candidates may wish to try to publish as they go. A doctoral study can be conceptualized as producing a series of publications. One does not need to limit oneself to publishing only when the findings are in and the study completed. There may be publishable papers arising from the literature review, the method, the findings and the discussion. Indeed, writing for publication will enhance your writing skills and may even help crystallize your arguments. There is obvious merit and value in having one's supervisor or academic adviser proof-read the sections as one writes them. In this way feedback and comments can be woven into the thesis as it develops. If writing this way, writing as one goes rather than at the end, it is quite possible that this will mean that the candidate actually writes more than one thesis! Yet the value in producing work that can be refined, developed and improved with the increasing academic, scholarly ability of the candidate as he or she progresses through the doctorate should not be underestimated. The 'pay-off' in terms of scholarship far outweighs any 'downside' in terms of additional writing workload.

Preparing to defend the thesis

Our basic edict for this chapter, namely that there is no one singular doctoral process, holds true for defending the thesis; there is no one singular correct way to offer an oral defence. However, there are some generic points which may assist in this preparation.

- Remember that no study is perfect (Cutcliffe and Stevenson, 2001). It is a laudable endeavour to attempt to produce the 'perfect' study, yet achieving this goal is unlikely. It is accepted as axiomatic that any study can always be improved and that all studies have limitations. Consequently, in offering an oral defence, be aware that you are not attempting to portray your study as perfect. This awareness leads logically onto the next point.
- Anticipate when to defend a point and when to concede a point. Your oral defence will need to be tempered by a degree of self-awareness. Particularly important is knowing which points to argue. It is well within the remit of the candidate to justify and argue his or her case. Indeed, the authors would expect this from the candidate as a demonstration of intellectual agility. However, a candidate who does not concede any limitation is likely to come across as a little arrogant and as lacking in awareness. Hence, candidates should be aware of when to concede and when to stand their ground.
- Know your study; anticipate questions regarding each constituent part of the thesis, e.g. literature review, methods, findings, discussion. As examiners, we would be wishing to see a deep and wide understanding from the candidate of each of the separate sections within his or her thesis and how these knit together. In fact, in examining theses, examiners often work their way through each section, highlight potential questions or issues and then systematically work through these during the oral defence. Hence, the well-prepared candidate will have a familiarity with each section and should expect questions pertaining to all these areas.
- Remember that the examiner is not trying to find fault with your study or with you! But they will expect you to be able to articulate substantive points, defend methodological decisions.
- It might be advantageous if the candidate can arrange to have a 'dry run' or 'rehearsal' of the oral defence. This can be arranged with the supervisor or academic adviser and there may even be facilities within the candidate's own academic department. This practice is not to equip the candidate with the answers which he or she can then regurgitate in the real oral. What it can do, however, is provide the candidate with a sense of what an oral defence can feel like, provide an insight into the types of questions that can be asked, reduce the candidate's anxiety that often surrounds a sense of the unknown.
- Lastly, there may be additional merit, particularly in terms of fielding awkward questions, if the candidate arranges to present his or her study to

one's departmental research colleagues at a research seminar or something similar. All these activities should increase the candidate's familiarity with both the content of their study and the experience of answering questions regarding their thesis.

Conclusion

In summary, undertaking doctoral education can be an arduous yet extremely rewarding activity. Not just rewarding in the final outcome but rewarding in the process of doing as well. It requires a conscious and deliberate decision to succeed; the adoption of a certain 'mind set' and commitment. Candidates need to be aware that undertaking doctoral education is a 'marathon' event rather than a 'sprint' and consequently is likely to have its high and low points. Such liability is normal; it should be expected and should not, in and of itself, discourage the candidate. While the authors would not subscribe to the position that upholds there being 'one' doctoral process, we have drawn on our own varied (and international) experiences in attempting to equip potential candidates with a number of strategies/tactics that may make for an increased chance of success. We wish you all well with your studies.

Notes

1 Often referred to colloquially as 'taught doctorates'.
2 Thus further indicating why one should not conceptualize 'the' doctoral process as a singular process.
3 The common if not preferred method for nurses in Canada, South Korea and the USA.
4 (And thus a good chance of attracting funding now and later.)
5 Evidence of this can be seen throughout government-led funding patterns within the UK in the past two decades. Recent examples include the research funding that was granted to studies which focused on HIV and AIDS, and more latterly on clinical supervision.
6 For example, if the candidate wishes to use grounded theory, then Glaser (1992) would strongly assert that the candidate have only a knowledge of the 'local concepts' and thus extensive literature reviews would not be appropriate.
7 This is especially the case with studies that have an emergent design.
8 For example, the University of Northern British Columbia offers doctoral candidates up to two-years-full time study leave at 60% salary. Plus, the candidate is encouraged to apply for 'top up' funding.
9 For example, medicine's historical preference and greater affinity for positivistic approaches, and psychiatric/mental health nurses' apparent comfort with qualitative approaches (Cutcliffe and Goward, 2000).
10 Sometimes, supervisors/academic advisers, funding bodies and examiners will check this process, and one cannot rely on memory or on *ad hoc* planning.
11 This is particularly important if you are doing a PhD by thesis, since this can be a lonely and/or isolated experience.
12 This can be addressed quite simply by constituting multidisciplinary graduate studies advisory committees.

References

Cutcliffe, J. R. and Goward, P. (2000). Mental health nurses and qualitative research methods: A mutual attraction? *Journal of Advanced Nursing,* **31**(3), 590–598.

Cutcliffe, J. R. and Stevenson, C. (2001). The long and winding road: Obtaining funding for qualitative research studies. *Nurse Researcher,* **9**(1), 52–63.

Cutcliffe, J. R. and Ward, M. (2003). *Critiquing nursing research.* London: Quay Books.

Glaser, B.G. (1992). *Basics of grounded theory analysis: Emergence vs forcing.* Mill Valley, CA: Sociological Press.

Glaser, B. G. (2001). *The Grounded Theory Perspective: Conceptualization Contrasted with Description.* Mill Valley, CA: Sociology Press.

Glaser, B.G. and Strauss A.L. (1967). *The discovery of grounded theory: strategies for qualitative research.* New York: Aldine Publ. Co.

McKenna, H. P., Cutcliffe, J. R., and McKenna, P. (2000). PhD or DNSc: What contribution to the substance of nursing? *All Ireland Journal of Nursing and Midwifery,* **1**(2), 55–59.

McKenna, H. P. and Cutcliffe, J. R. (2001). Nurse doctoral education in the United Kingdom and Ireland. *Online Journal of Issues in Nursing,* **5**(2), Manuscript 9. Available at: www.nursingworld.org/ojin/tpc12_9.htm (accessed on 27/06/04).

Morse, J. M. (1994). Designing funded qualitative research. In: N. K. Denzin, & Y. S. Lincoln (eds). *Handbook of qualitative research.* London: Sage, pp. 220–235.

Morse, J. M. and Field, P. A. (1994). *Qualitative research methods for health professionals.* 2nd edn. London: Sage.

Sandelowski, M. (1997). 'To be of use': Enhancing the utility of qualitative research. *Nursing Outlook,* **145**, 125–132.

Tripp-Reimer, T. and Cohen, M. Z. (1991). Funding strategies for qualitative research. In: J. M. Morse (ed.). *Qualitative research in nursing: A contemporary dialogue.* London: Sage, pp. 258–271.

van Manen, M. (2002). *Writing in the dark: Phenomenological studies in interpretive inquiry.* Ontario: Althouse Press.

Chapter 8

Role of the supervisor/mentor

Morag Gray and Callista Roy

Guiding and facilitating the development of students through their doctoral education and research experiences is a complex process which requires multiple skills and abilities. Whatever we call the person(s) involved in this challenging task, their understanding of the process can instil the required skills and their approaches can be improved with practice. Some may argue that ideally a research supervisor is synonymous with being a mentor. However, this is not always the case. There can be occasions where a research supervisor can be deemed to be a very good supervisor but for a variety of reasons the relationship does not develop into a lasting mentoring relationship.

Surprisingly, there is a dearth of published research on the actual supervision process of research students (Hawthorn, 1981; Bodley, 1991; Clifford, 1993; Sheehan, 1993; Marrow and Tatum 1994; Cottrell et al, 2002) and a few dissertations (Young, 1985; Alexander, 1986). However, there is much more research related to mentorship in general. Thus much of what is written in this chapter comes from experience, ours and others', and from extrapolations from related research studies.

Definitions

Research supervisor

If one compares the variety of roles expected of the mentor, in its classical sense, and that of a research supervisor, then there are a number of similarities. Barber and Norman (1987) define supervision as 'an interpersonal process where a skilled practitioner helps a less skilled practitioner to achieve professional abilities appropriate to his role. At the same time they are offered counsel and support' (p. 3). Howard and Sharp (1983) are more process-oriented in their definition of supervision. They assert that it contains two elements: advice seeking from the student and direction giving from the supervisor. Burnard and Morrison (1993) define supervision as 'the process through which one, more senior person, facilitates the growth and development of another colleague, in a professional and educational context' (p. 90).

Mentor

The term mentor originates from Homer's *Odyssey*. The detail of the accounts varies from author to author but essentially the story is as follows: Odysseus was the king of a small Greek island called Ithaca. He was married to Penelope and when their only son Telemachus was still an infant, the Trojan War began. Odysseus set off to fight in the Trojan War, which legend states lasted ten years. Before departing for the war, Odysseus appointed Mentor, who was an old and trusted friend, to be a tutor adviser to Telemachus and guardian to his estate (Butcher and Lang, 1883).

Confusion over the language used in association with mentorship in nursing has been identified for some time. Shapiro et al (1978) called for a clarification of concepts related to mentoring and even with repeated requests from others over the years, there has been no clear move forward (Merriam, 1983; Megel, 1985; Hagerty, 1986; Watts, 1986; Burnard, 1990; Donovan, 1990; Armitage and Burnard, 1991; Maggs, 1994; Woodrow, 1994). Authors have offered many different definitions and there is some consistency in the terms used to describe the mentor. Early work by Vance (1977) identified the classic mentor–protégé relationship as one in which an older, more experienced person guides, supports and nurtures a younger, less experienced one. Based on her study of nurse influentials, Vance added that the mentoring relationship involves a combination of behaviours and roles that contribute to both the professional and personal development of the protégé. Learning is enhanced by the mentor demonstrating the desired behaviour. The modelling influences are personalized by the mentor becoming directly involved with the protégé in a continuing relationship. In summary, Vance (1982) notes that a mentor may serve as a role model, guide, teacher, tutor, coach, confidant, and visionary-idealist.

Other authors offer similar perspectives of roles and behaviours. The mentor is older (Merriam, 1983; Burnard, 1988; Arnoldussen and White, 1990; Stachura and Hoff, 1990); more skilled and experienced than the person they mentor (Fagan and Fagan, 1983; Merriam 1983; Davis 1984; Darling 1985a; Burnard 1988; Hyde 1988; Foy and Waltho, 1989; Arnoldussen and White, 1990; Prestholdt, 1990; Brennan and Williams, 1993; DeMarco, 1993; Marshall, 1993); and wise and faithful (May et al, 1982; Megel 1985; Nyatanga and Bamford, 1990; Fields, 1991; Kelly, 1991).

A precise definition to which all can agree seems impossible. Prestholdt (1990) offers a definition that reflects the majority of opinion and research findings:

> Mentoring is viewed as a long term adult developmental process with active involvement in a close personal relationship. Mentors serve as counselors, teachers, sponsors, and guides for neophytes learning about their professions and how to cope with dynamic workplace realities.
>
> (Prestholdt, 1990 p. 26)

As Merriam (1983) states 'its meaning [mentor] appears to be defined by the scope of a research investigation or by a particular setting where it occurs' (p. 162). Hagerty (1986) concurs with Merriam's observation. Snelson et al (2002) state that 'the use of mentoring in many areas of nursing has been documented in the nursing literature such as the development of clinical practitioners, researchers and educators' (p. 655). It is therefore argued that the person(s) fulfilling the role could either be called a supervisor or mentor. Regardless of the title afforded the individual(s), what is vital is that the process takes place as effectively as possible.

Role and responsibilities of the supervisor/mentor

Anecdotal findings suggest that the role of the supervisor/mentor is diverse and multifaceted. Regardless of whether the term supervisor or mentor is used, in respect to the role, there are a number of similarities identified in the literature. These are listed in Table 8.1.

Brown and Atkins (1988) usefully link the role to aspects of research supervision which are identified below:

- Director (determining topic and method, providing ideas)
- Facilitator (providing access to resources or expertise, arranging fieldwork)
- Adviser (helping resolve technical problems, suggesting alternatives)
- Teacher (analysing possible research techniques and methods)
- Guide (suggesting table for writing up, giving feedback on progress, identifying critical path for data collection)
- Critic (providing feedback and direction on design of inquiry, of draft chapters, of interpretations of data)
- Freedom giver (authorizing student to make decisions, supporting student's decisions)
- Supporter (giving encouragement, showing interest, discussing student's ideas)
- Friend (extending interest and concern to non-academic aspects of student's life)
- Manager (checking progress regularly, monitoring study, giving systematic feedback, planning work)
- Examiner (such as suggesting internal examiner, mock vivas, interim progress reports, supervisory board member)

When contrasting the roles in Table 8.1 with aspects of research supervision by Brown and Atkins (1988), it can be seen that additional roles have been added which relate specifically to research supervision. As Brown and Atkins state 'given the range of possible roles it is not, perhaps, surprising that differences in opinion can exist as to what the role of the supervisor should be' (p. 120).

Table 8.1 Similarities in the role of the supervisor/mentor as described in the literature

Role	*Cited by*
Teacher	Kelly, 1978; Howard and Sharp, 1983; Merriam, 1983; Darling, 1984, 1985a; Armitage and Rees, 1988a; Davidhizar, 1988; Bracken and Davis, 1989; Northcott, 1989; Baker, 1990; Higginson, 1990; Prestholdt, 1990; Wright, 1990; Sloan and Slevin, 1991; Fields, 1991; Fox, 1991.
Supporter	Levinson, 1978; Merriam, 1983; Darling, 1984; Burnard, 1988; Davidhizar, 1988; Cahill and Kelly, 1989.
Encourager	Hawthorn, 1981; Davis, 1984; Burnard, 1988; Gottlieb, 1994.
An exemplar or role model	Levinson, 1978; May et al, 1982; Watts, 1986; Burnard, 1988; Cahill and Kelly, 1989; Baker, 1990; Wright, 1990; Kelly, 1991; Gottlieb, 1994, Zuber-Skerritt, 1994.
Counsellor	Levinson, 1978; Davis, 1984; Watts, 1986; Davidhizar, 1988; Cahill and Kelly, 1989; Northcott, 1989; Baker, 1990; Prestholdt, 1990; Fields, 1991; Kelly, 1991; Anforth, 1992.
Guide	Levinson, 1978; Hawthorn, 1981; Merriam, 1983; Darling, 1985a; Daloz, 1986; Watts, 1986; Armitage and Rees, 1988b; Cahill and Kelly, 1989; Foy and Waltho, 1989; Arnoldussen and White, 1990; Higginson, 1990; Prestholdt, 1990; Wright, 1990; Sloan and Slevin, 1991; Fields, 1991; Kelly, 1991; Anforth, 1992; Butterworth and Faugier, 1992; Williams and McLean, 1992; DeMarco, 1993; Marshall, 1993; Morton-Cooper and Palmer, 1993, 2000.
Adviser	Howard and Sharp, 1983; Merriam, 1983; Darling, 1985a; Armitage and Rees, 1988a, 1988b; Burnard, 1988; Laurent, 1988; Foy and Waltho, 1989; Northcott, 1989; Fields, 1991; Sloan and Slevin, 1991; Anforth, 1992.
Inspirer	Hawthorn, 1981; Darling, 1984; Burnard, 1988; Gottlieb, 1994.
Investor	Hawthorn, 1981; Darling, 1984; Gottlieb, 1994.
Trusted friend	Fagan and Fagan, 1983; Armitage and Rees, 1988b; Davidhizar, 1988; Fields, 1991; Anforth, 1992; Gottlieb, 1994.

Student's selection of a supervisor/mentor

Zhao (2001) reports that 'in the view of students, the ideal supervisor helps them to achieve a scientific, professional or personal goal, and to learn about research and how to conduct research against the quality standards of the system' (p. 2).

According to Brown and Atkins (1988) the most favourable qualities of a research supervisor/mentor were that the individual was knowledgeable, available, helpful and stimulating. Andersen and Shannon (1988) added that the chairperson's power and influence were the most significant and the primary socializing agent for doctoral candidates. Other characteristics to look for are experience with the system, an ability to give clear feedback and direction and to enhance the student's self-esteem. Zhao (2001) also adds clear guidance and parameters to the list. From a three-year longitudinal qualitative research study of student nurses, Gray and Smith (2000) identified the following qualities of an effective mentor: approachable; confident in their own ability; good communicator; professional; organized; enthusiastic, friendly, possessing a good sense of humour; caring; keen; enthusiastic; good role model; patient and understanding. These qualities can be easily attributed to that of an effective research supervisor. So these qualities should be uppermost in the mind of a student selecting a supervisor/mentor.

Choosing a supervisor is obviously important to the whole process, yet in many institutions, the supervisor is allocated by the head of the department (Phillips and Pugh, 2000). Higginson (1990) suggests that when considering the choice of supervisor, the less tangible qualities are the most important such as knowledge, enthusiasm, willingness and availability. She also warns to deliberate on the possibility of the supervisor retiring or leaving and ascertaining the arrangements which would be made in that instance. Higginson places the choice of the supervisor in equal importance to the choice of the research topic.

Phillips and Pugh (2000) suggest that the student ascertain whether their proposed supervisor has an established research record and is maintaining a contribution to the development of their field or discipline. An Association of American Colleges (AAC) report (1983) lists a number of questions that a newcomer can ask in looking for a mentor, including specifics such as: What panels and committees does the mentor serve on? What organizations does the mentor belong to and in what capacities? What influence does the mentor have in developing the discipline? Does the mentor know what is excellent in a given area and set high standards for self? Is the mentor someone who believes wholeheartedly in your abilities? What has happened to this person's former mentees in terms of positions, grants, and publications?

Sheehan (1993) contemplates the issue of choosing a supervisor against being matched or allocated. He concludes that there is no evidence available which indicates that one method is better than the other. For those who see supervision of research students assuming a mentorship quality, the mutual attraction of supervisor and student would be clearly important. That is to say the supervisor and the student would be kindred spirits. Indeed Sheehan (1993) cites research conducted by Elton and Pope (1989) in which they assert that the selection process 'should be one of matching students and supervisors for personal and academic compatibility, including the choice of the research topic' (p. 883). Sheehan (1993) himself concludes that a good match between supervisor and student is inherent in the supervisory process. Burnard and Morrison (1993) agree that this is the ideal situation.

Supervisor's/mentor's selection of a student

Delamont et al (1997) advise that when choosing a student one should reflect carefully on the skills and abilities a student requires in order to complete their doctoral studies: high level of motivation; ability to complete tasks (no previous false starts or abandoned courses); ability to work independently; evidence of intellectual creativity or at least some ideas of their own; ability to write and to be critical of previous work. In respect of mentors and mentees, Morton-Cooper and Palmer (2000) report that ideally, the two parties should be 'drawn together naturally by their personal characteristics, attributes and common values' (p. 41). Furthermore, Zhao (2001) states that one of the key issues derived from his study and supported by the literature is the 'matching of students and supervisors in terms of individual characteristics' (p. 4). The latter could be determined to some extent when interviewing doctoral candidates.

Experience and qualifications required by mentors

The experience and qualifications required by mentors are implied in the definition of the role and the discussion of selecting a mentor. Further, these will be specific to given programmes in particular settings. However, the qualifications for being a mentor for doctoral students can be explicated by examining some relevant documents on quality in doctoral education and work in progress on a position paper on mentoring by Roy et al (2003) for the International Network for Doctoral Education in Nursing. The following were examined to identify behaviours and capabilities desired for mentors: Pew Foundation project on Re-envisioning the PhD (2000); Indicators of quality in research-focused doctoral programmes in nursing (American Association of Colleges of Nursing [AACN] 2001); INDEN's Draft of quality indicators for doctoral programmes (INDEN, 2001); the University of Michigan handbooks on mentoring (Lewis, 2001) for both faculty and students; and work at the University of Maryland by Barbosa (2000). From these sources four categories were derived to include what is expected of a mentor: assistance, communication, guidance, and support. A 50-item opinionnaire was developed that included sections on qualifications, responsibilities, general expectations and expectations of students. Some relevant findings from piloting the opinionnaire with 14 faculty and 17 students from one doctoral programme in the USA are discussed below.

Faculty and students agreed that the following qualifications were *essential* for a mentor:

- a doctoral degree
- publication/recognition for research and scholarship
- awareness of the scope of the discipline and state of knowledge development and of a given area

- understanding of the programme and the procedure for approval of research.

Two items that more students than faculty felt were *essential* are experience and expertise related to the student's area of interest and experience in the guidance of research. Student comments included: 'The mentor should have been on enough committees' and should 'provide support and guidance; give the inside story and help interpret curriculum and policy; provide helpful feedback; open doors; be what one aspires to be and help students assimilate those characteristics' (Roy et al, 2003).

In relation to general expectations, faculty and students tended to agree in rating the following items as *essential* for a mentor:

- has a broad perspective on nursing as a discipline with a specific focus of research interests that leads to significant contributions to knowledge for nursing
- has a commitment to the sustained time and effort required of a scholar and mentor in nursing
- ensures the responsible conduct of science
- has a record of fulfilling scholarly and academic commitments in a timely fashion
- is committed to the student's success and completion of the programme in a reasonable time period
- is competent in research writing and capable of directing others in developing these skills.

Both groups were close to evenly split between the following two items as *essential* or *preferable:*

- is actively involved in the key issues and debates of nursing as a scholarly discipline
- maintains a network of contacts who can be called upon as resources for student.

One faculty comment at the end of this section asked whether 'mentors must get mentored'. One student noted that the student needed self-direction and initiative and to not be dependent.

The identification of consensus within a given school and follow-up faculty development programmes can lead to better understanding of the process of mentoring and to the enhancement of the skills and abilities needed (Roy et al, 2003).

Nature of the student–supervisor/mentor relationship

The nature of the relationship between student and supervisor/mentor is crucial to the successful submission of a doctoral thesis. It is vital that a trusting working relationship is established as early as possible. This can be achieved through setting and agreeing upon ground rules from the onset, as it is from this process that each party is able to explore what their expectations are and arrange a set of guidelines on which there is mutual agreement (Delamont et al, 1997; Zhao, 2001).

Armitage and Rees (1988a) counsel that it is imperative that each party is aware of their respective roles and functions, and they suggest that a worthwhile strategy is the creation of a verbal or written contract. The contract should cover time frames, agreements over deadlines, minimum number of supervision hours which will be offered, and the ethical and administrative aspects of the research (Armitage and Rees, 1988a; Ryan, 1994), and should be detailed to avoid supervision problems arising from lack of clarity (Phillips, 1994; Ryan, 1994). Johns (1994) discussed the construction of contracts in relation to reflective practice, and offered a rationale for contract setting: 'Contracting sets the stage for a relationship built on trust; a climate of trust being essential to enable the practitioner to feel free to share her experiences without a fear of being judged' (p. 120). This would seem an admirable motivation for using contracts within research supervision. Contracts should be reviewed on a regular basis. Ryan (1994) suggests informally every three months and formally every six months.

The rationale for reviewing the contract or agreed guidelines is that over time, the nature of the relationship changes. In earlier work Young (1985) noted that the protégé's perception of the conflict resolution process in different phases of the relationship was a crucial element in the ability to grow and develop from the relationship. Morton-Cooper and Palmer (2000) suggest that over time students gradually gain in confidence and develop the capacity to 'go it alone'. They cite Hunt and Mitchell's (1993) four-stage model which involves initiation, training, termination and the formation of an amicable ending of the supervision process with the establishment of a peer friendship. Supervisors need to be good listeners and be able to create an environment conducive to the student sharing problems or difficulties (Armitage and Rees, 1988a; van Ooijen, 1994). They also need to be highly interested in the research in order to inspire their student (Clifford, 1993).

In discussing a role relationship that is complex and multidimensional in relation to both skills and personal qualities, it may be useful to list the frequently quoted 12 strategies for effective mentoring published by Noller (1982).

- Positive attitude: encourage the mentee to approach life and goals with enthusiasm and to be accepting of self and others.
- Valuing: encourage a person to examine beliefs and ideals in an effort to establish personal values and goals.

- Open-mindedness: encourage a person to keep an open mind to ideas.
- Interrelations: the interactions between mentor and mentee should be situations of sharing, caring and empathizing.
- Creative problem solving: encourage the mentee to use a creative problem-solving process.
- Effective communication: encourage a person to be an attentive listener and an assertive questioner.
- Discovery: encourage the mentee to be an independent thinker.
- Strengths and uniqueness: encourage a person to recognize individual strengths and uniqueness and to build on them.
- Confidence: assist a person in developing self-confidence.
- Awareness: stress that an individual be aware of the environment, be intuitive, be problem sensitive, and be ready to make the most of opportunities.
- Risk-taking: encourage a person to be a risk-taker and to be an active participant, not a spectator.
- Flexibility: share with a mentee the importance of being flexible and adaptable in attitudes and actions, looking for alternatives, and seeing situations/persons from different perspectives.

The process

The aim of the process is to enhance the student's knowledge, skills and ability to conduct research (Zhao, 2001). The main features of the process are reassurance and motivation to maintain the student's confidence and enthusiasm (Delamont et al, 1997); these authors highlight that feedback on progress is essential as without it students are unlikely to progress. Brown and Atkins (1988) maintain that the process should take place in a safe and relaxed environment in which regular, planned and structured work outputs are established and agreed to.

Perhaps the most critical aspect is the management of time. Completing a PhD full time generally takes three years and part time five years. This may seem a long time to the research student but from experience the supervisor knows the dangers of allowing the student to adopt a false sense of security. Phillips and Pugh (2000) are of the opinion that students should never underestimate the amount of time the process takes. Supervisors should therefore get the student to work out a timetable of events and set realistic deadlines. Phillips and Pugh (2000) counsel to ensure that holidays (both students' and supervisors') are entered into a timetable as these are often missed. Although the supervisor will give advice and guidance on the suitability of the timetable, it must be made clear to the student that it is they who are in control of their research and not their supervisor.

The issue of establishing time frames and deadlines has been discussed by several authors (Armitage and Rees, 1988a, 1988b; Sheehan, 1993; Brown, 1994; Phillips and Pugh, 2000). Sheehan (1993) cites the work of Welsh (1981) who used a small sample of 37 PhD students to discover that one of the most important features of completing their studies was organization. Since it was a small study, it is inappropriate to generalize the findings but there is anecdotal evidence to support Welsh's findings (Armitage and Rees, 1988a).

Brown (1994) and Phillips and Pugh (2000) give advice regarding timetables. The student should work backwards from the submission date and set deadlines for specific stages in the research. Incorporated within the deadlines should be target dates for completion of writing. Brown (1994) in particular is most insistent that deadlines once set are non-negotiable; both parties should abide by them. Where Brown (1994) will not tolerate flexibility within the time frames, Armitage and Rees (1988a, 1988b) believe that the emphasis should be on developing a realistic timetable and argue that a flexible approach is a strength rather than a weakness.

Zhao (2001) offers a supervision plan (Table 8.2) from defining the research topic to the final stage of thesis writing. Performance indicators are incorporated within the plan as a means of establishing goals to meet benchmarks of best practices.

Table 8.2 'Supervision plan for PhD candidature (Zhao 2001, p. 7)'

Research process/milestone	*Supervision process*
• Defining research topic/problem • Developing research methodology, theoretical framework • Designing research • Conducting literature review • Collecting data • Analysing/interpreting data • Writing thesis	• Facilitating students' access to knowledge, information, database • Creating knowledge repositories through guiding students to present and publish their work • Enhance knowledge/research environment through facilitating students' networking and sharing knowledge/research • Embedding knowledge in the students and their thesis
Performance indicator	*Timeline (equivalent full-time)*
• A right match of supervisor and student • Level of effectiveness in providing guidance to students • Quality and timeliness of meetings and interaction • Extent of relevance and appropriateness of assessment and feedback given to students • Level of adherence to pre-set project objectives • Milestones achieved in the planned time	• 6–12 months (research proposal) • 3–6 months (literature review) • 12–18 months (collecting/analysing/interpreting data) • 9–12 months (writing thesis) **Total:** 30 months (minimum) 48 months (maximum)

Benefits of the mentoring process

The benefits of the mentoring process for the protégé are apparent, including advice and information to complete the doctoral research. Also indirect benefits may accrue through the mentor's own connections and contacts. For example, the mentor can introduce the protégé to key scholars in the field, can talk about the protégé's research to senior colleagues, and nominate the protégé for awards or prizes. The mentor can give specific advice on what organizations and conferences are most important and can help the protégé get on a given programme. More generally, a deeper sense of commitment to the role of scholar is often gained through the mentoring process.

The relationship offers benefits for the mentor as well. There is satisfaction in helping to create a scholar who can carry on work in the field. Specifically, the mentor receives feedback on projects from a person who is eager to learn and committed to the success of the mentor's work. The mentor finds that her or his own network of colleagues, visibility and influence expands as protégés accept positions at other institutions and some return to their own countries.

According to the AAC report (1983) referred to earlier, there are also benefits for the institution from mentoring processes. Effective mentoring contributes to scholarly productivity and commitment. There is less attrition of both students and faculty as cooperation and cohesiveness are encouraged in mentoring relationships. Providing skills for success makes graduates ambassadors of positive attitudes for the institution.

Challenges arising during the mentoring process

During the supervision/mentoring process challenges and difficulties arise that both parties need to understand and address. Anecdotal evidence suggests that problems may include reluctance of the student to accept less support and guidance from the supervisor as the study progresses (Phillips and Pugh, 2000), boredom and lack of motivation (Howard and Sharp, 1983; Grant and Graham, 1994; Phillips and Pugh, 2000), frustration, a desire to get it finished, not keeping to the timetable (Phillips and Pugh, 2000), and dissatisfaction with the supervision given (Grant and Graham, 1994). This is often related to an unrealistic expectation on the part of the student, for as Burnard and Morrison (1993) and Grant and Graham (1994) explain, whereas the research is at the centre of the student's life, the student is only one of the many facets of the supervisor's life.

Nelson and Friedlander (2001) conducted a qualitative research study with the aim of investigating negative research supervision. They interviewed 13 Master's and doctoral students. Their findings indicated that problems principally arose from a poor relationship between supervisor and student, with the students reporting excessive levels of stress and self-doubt; ongoing power struggles with their supervisor and the need to rely on peers, and other professionals and therapists for support. Similarly, Young (1985) noted the protégé's perception of the need for conflict resolution for growth in the relationship.

Darling (1985b) describes what she calls a gallery of toxic mentors: avoiders; dumpers; blockers; and destroyers/criticizers. Avoiders make themselves scarce when it comes to having anything to do with the student. Wilson-Barnett et al (1995) call this type of toxic mentor an 'absent mentor'. An example would be a supervisor who consistently changes agreed appointments for meetings or generally make herself unavailable or unapproachable. Dumpers, according to Darling (1985b), have the deliberate philosophy of throwing students in at the deep end, hoping that they swim in the process. Dumpers literally abdicate all responsibility for the student. An example would be the supervisor who pushes the student into doing things before they felt ready or forces them into doing things for which they can see no relevance. Blockers are individuals who refuse to meet the student's needs. They can do this in three ways. They can positively refuse (refuser) to help the student, for example, telling them that they can learn that later. They can deliberately withhold (withholder) information, knowledge and skills. Lastly, blockers can inhibit the student's development by too close supervision (hoverer). An example of the latter would be a supervisor who failed to allow the student to 'acquire those techniques and methods themselves without stultifying or warping their own intellectual development' (Brown and Atkins, 1988, p. 115). Destroyers/criticizers are described by Darling (1985b) as working either subtly as underminers or more overtly as criticizers or belittlers.

Brown and Atkins (1988, p. 123) list the common problems affecting research students as:

- poor planning and management of project
- methodological difficulties in the research
- writing-up
- isolation
- personal problems outside the research
- inadequate or negligent supervision.

Brown and Atkins (1988, p. 127) also list the common criticisms of supervisors as:

- too few meetings with students
- no interest in student
- no interest in topic
- too little practical help given
- too little direction
- failure to return work promptly
- absence from department
- lack of research experience
- lack of relevant skills and/or knowledge.

The use of multiple mentors offered by (AAC, 1983) is described as one way to deal with the problems that arise in direct one-to-one mentoring relationships. Short-term mentors for specific skills and advice may be appropriate. Accepting weak ties for specific advice, guidance, and support from on and off campus at various stages may be effective. The novice also needs to be aware that the search for the perfect mentor may be futile. Every organization should provide guidelines related to sexual attractions within mentoring relationships. Most university campuses today have well publicized policies and procedures to deal with the general area of sexual harassment.

International collaboration and networking among colleagues for mentor development

The crucial and multifaceted process of the supervision of research students is an area long overdue for research. It seems somewhat inconsistent that supervisors demand rigour when conducting research and the use of empirical evidence to back up actions, and yet the process used in the actual mechanism of supervision is mainly based on anecdotal, experiential findings, and a small number of qualitative studies. Further, Vance (1982) notes that the two theories that are used in research studies on mentoring are Erikson's (1963, 1968) developmental stage of generativity and Bandura's (1977) social learning theory. Grand- and mid-range theories in nursing provide possibilities for the design of studies specific to mentoring in nursing. Examples are: Peplau's theory of interpersonal relationships (1994), Roy's theories of self concept, role function, and interdependence (1976), Meleis and others' work on transitions (2000), and Reed's self-transcendence theory (1989).

It is therefore recommended that an international collaborative research study be undertaken grounded on a given theoretical basis that provides for conceptual and empirical definitions of terms. Such a study could clarify the meaning and processes of mentoring and provide guidance for the development of successful mentoring.

Recognizing that practising mentoring improves one's abilities, we face some particular problems. Some countries are facing faculty shortages due to retirement of experienced senior faculty and in other geographic areas, the preparation of mentors cannot keep pace with the need. The AAC (1983) notes that successful women mentors are most likely to be over-used. Creative use of retired faculty as mentors to the mentors through electronic chat rooms is another possibility to extend the expertise and wisdom needed.

When international students are involved, it is recommended that particular attention be given to the mentoring relationship. Meleis (2003) suggests being in touch with key persons in the country of origin to share key events of the visiting student; having welcoming events and other strategies to make these students feel an important part of the community of scholars; and drawing on their knowledge and expertise from their home countries. For example, one school is having an annual celebration of unity and diversity planned around a USA-style Christmas party that will allow international students to share their differing cultural and religious beliefs.

On the local level, it is recommended that within universities specific processes be instituted to come to some consensus on the process of mentoring and that faculty be encouraged to share successful strategies as well as issues that arise. The International Network for Doctoral Education in Nursing is taking leadership in providing materials and processes for individual schools, and for a broader dialogue that can strengthen the important process of mentoring doctoral students.

References

Association of American Colleges (AAC) (1983). *Academic mentoring for women students and faculty: A new look at an old way to get ahead.* Project on the Status and Education of Women, Association of American Colleges.Washington, DC: AAC.

American Association of Colleges of Nursing (AACN) (2001). *Indicators of quality in research-focused doctoral programs in nursing.* Washington, DC: AACN.

Alexander, D. W. (1986). An investigation of deans' perceptions of attributes present in the mentor/mentee relationship [Doctoral dissertation, University of Texas at Austin]. *Dissertation Abstracts International*, **47**, 3703B.

Anderson, E.M. and Shannon, A.L. (1988). Toward a conceptualisation of mentoring. *Journal of Teacher Education*, **39**(1), 38–42.

Anforth, P. (1992). Mentors, not assessors. *Nurse Education Today,* **12**(4), 299–302.

Armitage, P. and Burnard, P. (1991). Mentors or preceptors? Narrowing the theory-practice gap. *Nurse Education Today,* **11**(3), 225–229.

Armitage, S. and Rees, C. (1988a). Project supervision. *Nurse Education Today,* **8**, 99–104.

Armitage, S. and Rees, C. (1988b). Student projects: A practical framework. *Nurse Education Today*, **8**, 289–295.

Arnoldussen, B. and White, L. M. (1990). The mentoring experience. *Nursing Administration Quarterly,* **15**(1), 28–35.

Baker, S. (1990). The key to nurse education? *Nursing Standard,* **4**(39), 43.

Bandura, A. (1977). *Social learning theory*. Englewood Cliffs, NJ: Prentice-Hall.

Barber, P. and Norman, L. (1987). Skills in supervision. *Nursing Times,* **83**(2), 3–4.

Barbosa, P. (2000). Strengthening your graduate program through mentorship. Available at: www.gradschool.umed.edu/mentorship/mentorexpect.htm/ (accessed on 14.04.2002).

Bodley, D. E. (1991). Adapting supervision strategies to meet the challenges of future mental health nursing practice. *Nurse Education Today,* **11**, 378–386.

Bracken, E. and Davis, J. (1989). The implications of mentorship in nursing career development. *Senior Nurse,* **9**(5), 15–16.

Brennan, A. and Williams, D. (1993). Preceptorship: Is it a workable concept? *Nursing Standard,* **7**(52), 34–36.

Brown, G. and Atkins, M. (1988). *Effective teaching in higher education.* London: Kogan Page.

Brown, R. (1994). The 'Big Picture' about managing writing. In: O. Zuber-Skerritt and Y. Ryan (eds). *Quality in Postgraduate Education*. London: Kogan Page.

Burnard, P. (1988). A supporting act. *Nursing Times*, **84**(46), 27–28.

Burnard, P. (1990). The student experience: Adult learning and mentorship revisited. *Nurse Education Today*, **10**(5), 349–354.

Burnard, P. and Morrison, P. (1993). *Survival guide for nursing students*. Oxford: Butterworth Heinemann.

Butcher, S. H. and Lang, A. (1883). *The Odyssey of Homer*. 4th edn. London: Macmillan & Co.

Butterworth, T. and Faugier, J. (1992). *Clinical supervision and mentorship in nursing*. London: Chapman and Hall.

Cahill, M. F. and Kelly, J. J. (1989). A mentor program for nursing majors. *Journal of Nursing Education*, **28**(1), 40–42.

Clifford, C. (1993). The role of nurse teachers in the empowerment of nurses through research. *Nurse Education Today*, **13**, 47–54.

Cottrell, D., Kilminister, S., Jolly, B. and Grant, J. (2002). What is effective supervision and how does it happen? A critical incident study. *Medical Education*, **36**, 1042–1049.

Daloz, L. A. (1986). *Effective teaching and mentoring*. San Francisco, CA: Jossey-Bass.

Darling, L. A. W. (1984). What do nurses want in a mentor? *The Journal of Nursing Administration*, **14**(10), 42–44.

Darling, L. A. W. (1985a). Mentors and mentoring. *Nurse Educator*, **10**(6), 18–19.

Darling, L. A. W. (1985b). What to do about toxic mentors. *Journal of Nursing Administration*, **15**(5), 43–44.

Davidhizar, R. E. (1988). Mentoring in doctoral education. *Journal of Advanced Nursing*, **13**(6), 775–781.

Davis, A. J. (1984). You need someone older and wiser. *American Journal of Nursing*, **84**(10), 1290–1291.

Delamont, S., Atkinson, P. and Parry, O. (1997). *Supervising the PhD: A guide to success*. Buckingham: Open University Press.

DeMarco, R. (1993). Mentorship: A feminist critique of current research. *Journal of Advanced Nursing*, **18**(8), 1242–1250.

Donovan, J. (1990). The concept and role of mentor. *Nurse Education Today*, **10**, 294–298.

Elton, L. and Pope, M. (1989). Research supervision: The value of collegiality. *Cambridge Journal of Education*, **19**(3), 267–276.

Erikson, E. (1963). *Childhood and society*. New York, NY: Norton.

Erikson, E. H., Piaget, J. and Sears, R. R. (1966). *Three theories of child development*. New York, NY: Harper Row.

Erikson, E. (1968). *Identity: Youth and crisis*. New York, NY: Norton.

Fagan, M. M. and Fagan, P. D. (1983). Mentoring among nurses. *Nursing and Health Care*, **4**, 77–82.

Fields, W. L. (1991). Mentoring in nursing: A historical approach. *Nursing Outlook*, **39**(6), 257–261.

Fox, J. (1991). Mentorship and the charge nurse. *Nursing Standard*, **5**(23), 34–36.

Foy, H. and Waltho, B. J. (1989). The mentor system: Are learner nurses benefiting? *Senior Nurse*, **9**(5), 24–25.

Gottlieb, N. (1994). Supervising the writing of a thesis. In: O. Zuber-Skerritt and Y. Ryan (eds). *Quality in Postgraduate Education*. London: Kogan Page.

Grant, B. and Graham, A. (1994). Guidelines for discussion: A tool for managing postgraduate supervision. In: O. Zuber-Skerritt and Y. Ryan (eds). *Quality in Postgraduate Education*. London: Kogan Page.

Gray, M. A. and Smith, L. N. (2000). The qualities of an effective mentor from the student nurse's perspective: Findings from a longitudinal qualitative study. *Journal of Advanced Nursing*, **32**(6), 1542–1549.

Hagerty, B. (1986). A second look at mentors. *Nursing Outlook*, **34**(1), 16–24.

Hawthorn, P. J. (1981). Supervision of dissertations of undergraduate nursing students. *Nursing Times*, 77(5), 29–30.

Higginson, I. (1990). Research degree supervision: Lottery or life belt. *Critical Public Health*, **3**, 42–47.

Howard, K. and Sharp, J. A. (1983). *The management of a student research project*. Hampshire: Gower.

Hunt, D. and Mitchell, C. (1993). Mentorship. A career training development tool. *Academy of Management Review*, **3**, 475–485.

Hyde, J. (1988). *A Guide to the role of the mentor*. London: Royal College of Nursing.

International Network for Doctoral Education in Nursing: Task Force on Quality (2001). *International quality criteria and indicators for doctoral programs*. Presented in Copenhagen, Denmark.

Johns, C. (1994). Guided reflection. In: A. Palmer, S. Burns and C. Bulman (eds). *Reflective practice in nursing. The growth of the professional practitioner*. Oxford: Blackwell Scientific.

Kelly, L. Y. (1978). Power guide – the mentor relationship. *Nursing Outlook*, **26**, 339.

Kelly, L. Y. (1991). *Dimensions of professional nursing*. New York, NY: Pergamon Press.

Laurent, C. (1988). On hand to help. *Nursing Times*, **84**(46), 29–30.

Levinson, D. (1978). *The seasons of a man's life*. New York, NY: Ballantine.

Lewis, E. (ed.) (2001). *How to get the mentoring you want: A guide for graduate students at a diverse university*. University of Michigan Press. Available from www.rackham.umich.edu/studentinfo/publications/studentmentoring/contents.html (accessed 04.2002).

Maggs, C. (1994). Mentorship in nursing and midwifery education: issues for research. *Nurse Education Today*, **14**(1), 22–29.

Marrow, C. E. and Tatum, S. (1994). Student supervision: Myth or reality. *Journal of Advanced Nursing*, **19**, 1247–1255.

Marshall, C. (1993). Mentorship in critical care. *British Journal of Theatre Nursing*, **2**(11), 22–23.

May, K. M., Meleis, A. I. and Winstead-Fry, P. (1982). Mentorship for scholarliness: Opportunities and dilemmas. *Nursing Outlook*, **30**(1), 22–28.

Megel, M. E. (1985). New faculty in nursing: Socialization and the role of the mentor. *Journal of Nursing Education*, **24**(7), 303–306.

Meleis, A., Sawyer, L., Im, E. et al (2000). Experiencing transitions: An emerging middle-range theory. *Advances in Nursing Science* **23**, 12–28.

Meleis, A. I. (2003). International students: Trends and challenges. Presentation at AACN 2003 Doctoral Education Conference, January, Sanibel Island, FL.

Merriam, S. (1983). Mentors and proteges: A critical review of the literature. *Adult Education Quarterly*, **33**(3), 161–173.

Morton-Cooper, A. and Palmer, A. (1993). *Mentoring and preceptorship. A guide to support roles in clinical practice*. Oxford: Blackwell Scientific.

Morton-Cooper, A. and Palmer, A. (2000). *Mentoring and preceptorship. A guide to support roles in clinical practice.* 2nd edn. Oxford: Blackwell Scientific.

Nelson, M. L. and Friedlander, M. L. (2001). A close look at conflictual supervisory relationships: The trainee's perspective. *Journal of Counseling Psychology,* **48**(4), 384–395.

Noller, R. B. (1982). Mentoring: A renaissance of apprenticeship. *The Journal of Creative Behavior,* **16**(1), 1–4.

Northcott, N. (1989). Mentorship in nurse education. *Nursing Standard,* 3(24), 25–28.

Nyatanga, L. and Bamford, M. (1990). Mentorship scheme using the experiential taxonomy (ET). *Senior Nurse,* **10**(5), 14–15.

Peplau, H.E. (1994). *Interpersonal theory in nursing.* Basingstoke, UK: Macmillan.

Phillips, E. (1994). Avoiding communication breakdown. In: O. Zuber-Skerritt and Y. Ryan (eds). *Quality in Postgraduate Education.* London: Kogan Page.

Phillips, E. M. & Pugh, D. S. (2000). *How to get a PhD.* 3rd edn. Milton Keynes: Open University Press.

Prestholdt, C. O. (1990). Modern mentoring: strategies for developing contemporary nursing leadership. *Nursing Administration Quarterly,* **15**(1), 20–27.

Reed, P. G. (1989). Nursing theorizing as an ethical endeavor. *Advances in Nursing Science* **11**(3), 109.

Re-envisioning the PhD. Meta-themes from the National Conference. Center for Instructional Development and Research, University of Washington (2000). http://www.grad.washington.edu/envision/project_resources/metathemes.html (accessed 14.05.2004).

Roy, C. (1976). *Introduction to nursing: An adaptation model.* Englewood Cliffs, NJ: Prentice-Hall.

Roy, C., Murphy, M. and Eisenhauer, L. (2003). Mentoring: A project in process. *INDEN Newsletter,* **2**(3), 3–7.

Ryan, Y. (1994). Contracts and checklists: Practical propositions for postgraduate supervision. In: O. Zuber-Skerritt and Y. Ryan (eds). *Quality in Postgraduate Education.* London: Kogan Page.

Shapiro, E. C. Haseltine, F. P. and Rowe, M. P. (1978). Moving up: Models, mentors, and the 'Patron system'. *Sloan Management Review,* **19**(3), 51–58.

Sheehan, J. (1993). Issues in the supervision of postgraduate research students in nursing. *Journal of Advanced Nursing,* **18**(6), 880–885.

Sloan, J.P. and Slevin, O. (1991). *Teaching and supervision of student nurses during practice placements.* Belfast, NI: National Board for Nursing, Midwifery and Health Visiting for Northern Ireland.

Snelson, C. M., Martsolf, D. S. and Dieckman, B. C., (2002). Caring as a theoretical perspective for a nursing faculty mentoring program. *Nurse Education Today,* **22**, 654–660.

Stachura, L. M. and Hoff, J. (1990). Toward achievement of mentoring for nurses. *Nursing Administration Quarterly,* **15**(1), 56–62.

Vance, C. N. (1977). A group profile of contemporary influentials in American nursing. [Doctoral dissertation, Teachers College, Columbia Univeristy]. *Dissertation Abstracts International,* **38**, 4734B.

Vance, C. N. (1982). The mentor connection. *The Journal of Nursing Administration,* **12**(4), 7–13.

van Ooijen, E. (1994). Whipping up a storm. *Nursing Standard,* **16**(9), 48.

Watts, A. G. (1986). 'Mentoring.' *Counselling,* **57**(August), 4–7.

Welsh, J. M. (1981). The PhD student at work. *Studies in Higher Education*, **6**(2), 159–162.

Williams, B. and McLean, I. (1992). Someone to turn to. *Nursing Times*, **88**(38), 48–49.

Wilson-Barnett, J., Butterworth, T., White, E. et al (1995). Clinical support and the Project 2000 nursing student: Factors influencing this process. *Journal of Advanced Nursing*, **21**, 1152–1158.

Woodrow, P. (1994). Mentorship: Perceptions and pitfalls for nursing practice. *Journal of Advanced Nursing*, **19**(5), 812–818.

Wright, C. M. (1990). An innovation in a diploma program: The future potential of mentorship in nursing. *Nurse Education Today*, **10**, 355–359.

Young, C. F. (1985). Women as protégés: The perceptual development of female doctoral students who have completed their initial mentor-protégé relationship. [Doctoral dissertation, Syracuse University]. *Dissertation Abstracts International*, 47, 1903A.

Zhao, F. (2001). Postgraduate research supervision: A process of knowledge management. http://www2.cddc.vt.edu/ultibase/Articles/may01/zhao1.htm (accessed on 07.07.03).

Zuber-Skerritt, O. (1994). Improving the quality of postgraduate supervision through residential staff development programmes. In: O. Zuber-Skerritt and Y. Ryan (eds). *Quality in postgraduate education*. London: Kogan Page.

Chapter 9

Quality monitoring and quality criteria for doctoral programmes: a global perspective

Mi Ja Kim, Jenifer Wilson-Barnett and Rosalina A. P. Rodrigues

The mission of doctoral programmes is to train researchers with the critical and reflective capacity for the development of scientific knowledge. Nursing scholarship values connection to practice, substantive mastery of nursing areas, philosophical analyses, rigorous investigations, and a social awareness of the relationship between knowledge development and impact on society, among others (Meleis et al, 1994).

Doctoral programmes in nursing have enjoyed rapid growth in many countries in recent decades. While this is a positive sign for the advancement of nursing science, many nurse educators and scholars worldwide have been increasingly concerned about the quality of doctoral education, particularly regarding the quality of the programmes, the faculty and their research, the students, and the institutional resources and infrastructure to support doctoral education. This sentiment was aptly echoed by Anderson (2000), who emphasized the importance of ensuring appropriate prescribed standards for doctoral degrees, given the rapid growth of academic nursing in many Western countries. Minnick and Halstead (2002) noted in their survey of 87 doctoral programmes in the USA the importance of having consensus among doctoral educators if we are to improve the quality of doctoral education.

In the past decade, quality assurance has become more formalized; previously, arrangements were often informal and quality depended on individual supervisors (Pearson, 1996). However, the operationalization of standard statements for quality assurance in doctorates has challenged many universities in the UK (Schmitt, 1999). The same can be said about Brazil and the USA.

This chapter describes the major components of quality in doctoral programmes and quality monitoring and evaluation processes from the perspectives of Brazil, the UK and the USA. Since each country has a different educational system and uses different terminologies for similar roles and functions, comparable words are added by '/' wherever applicable, while preserving the unique features of the countries.

Components of quality in doctoral programmes

Mission of institution/university and quality of doctoral programmes

The quality of doctoral education is largely dictated by the mission of the university in which the nursing programme resides. Doctoral degree granting universities are usually research intensive with the tripartite mission of teaching, research and service. In keeping with this mission, nursing doctoral programmes usually place major emphasis on research, although the curriculum varies across countries. For instance, most doctoral programmes (including PhD or DNS [Doctorate of Nursing Science] degree programmes) in the USA and Brazil have both coursework and research training, whereas, in Europe, many doctoral programmes do not have any coursework. Elements for formal courses usually include nursing theory, philosophy of science, advanced research methods, statistics, research and theory in areas of nursing science, and cognate areas related to the nursing investigation. Other courses or informal teachings focus on analytical and leadership strategies for dealing with social, ethical, cultural, economic and political issues related to nursing and health care. The introduction of more taught components/coursework across many countries has also highlighted the need to make research training more sophisticated and comprehensive (Pearson, 1999).

The type of doctoral programme also determines the curriculum. PhD programmes primarily focus on research training, whereas professional doctoral degree programmes (such as DNS) focus primarily on professional practice issues. However, there are few differences between the two programmes in the USA, as found by the American Association of Colleges of Nursing (2001): 'The content and course requirements may vary slightly and the emphasis may be on empirical versus applied research, but the focus of the programme is to prepare students to pursue intellectual inquiry and conduct independent research for the purpose of extending knowledge' (p. 7). The similarities come from the historical development of doctoral programmes in nursing within the university systems in the USA; both types of degree programmes require university approval; however, the PhD operates under the aegis of the graduate school, while the DNS does not.

In Brazil, the quality of doctoral programmes is governed by the graduate guidelines set by the Foundation Coordination for the Improvement of Higher Education Personnel (*Fundação Coordenação de Aperfeiçoamento de Pessoal de Nível Superior [CAPES]*). This is a sponsoring agency that supports the Ministry of Education and Culture (MEC/CAPES, 2002). For instance, CAPES coordinates the training of human resources by accrediting and re-accrediting graduate programmes. There are norms established by Sucupira Resolutions 977/65 and 77/69 of the Federal Education Council for creating doctoral programmes in nursing to train researchers. The Lash study's (1992) finding that institutional quality (particularly that of graduate programmes) greatly affects postdoctoral career attainment highlights our responsibility to uphold the quality of doctoral programmes in nursing for the success of our graduates' careers.

Faculty expertise and responsibilities

In many countries, nursing PhDs are still relatively small in number, although growth has been rapid. This small number is reflected in the number of faculty with doctoral degrees. In the USA, less than 50% of nursing faculty in baccalaureate and higher degree programmes possess doctorates (Anderson, 2000). This number may have improved somewhat, but this clearly indicates that we not only have to accelerate the number of doctorally-prepared faculty, but also focus on faculty development activities for teaching and advising doctoral students, especially if other countries experience a similar situation. To prepare faculty/academic staff who supervise PhDs in the UK, faculty members with new PhD degrees in the past became co-supervisors/advisers for one or two students and then became main supervisors/major advisers. However, there is increasing realization that a more structured team approach with at least two supervisors is required with regular reporting schedules and formalized preparation for supervisors. This may include faculty from other disciplines, as greater confidence may be generated across faculties and for individual supervisors. Guidance also exists for joint supervision/advisement, if it becomes necessary. In addition, training courses exist in most universities with the edict that all supervisors should have this formal assessment. Observing PhD vivas (final oral defence of the dissertation) is also one of the best learning opportunities for all supervisors, providing that candidates do not object.

Preparation for supervisors/faculty advisers should include workshops, regular faculty meetings, membership of PhD review panels/the graduate faculty, collegial mentoring, and co-supervision for more than two students. Skills in supervision include the ability to promote intellectual growth in students, appropriate knowledge of up-to-date literature and information technology (IT) search engines, access to a network of other academics and experts, and a familiarity and hopefully partnerships with health services colleagues. Clearly, sophisticated understanding of research methodology used in the PhD study is essential, and constant attendance at relevant conferences and updating of methodological developments should ensure this is maintained.

Academic staff/faculty expertise to supervise students and ensuring that PhD programmes are educationally rewarding are important aspects of faculty advisers to make the experience of undertaking a PhD not too stressful or isolating and to assure that the goal of a PhD leads to career gains and personal fulfilment.

Matching subject areas for students and supervisers/faculty advisers is challenging, particularly in smaller institutions. This has led topic areas to be more focused and academics/faculty members and students to be more selective and careful in choosing supervisors/faculty advisers. Greater access to information via the World Wide Web and Internet sites means that academics/faculty can promote their fields of expertise and previous work. This enables prospective students to 'shop around.' Less mobile candidates may select supervisors/faculty advisers through personal contact or through a more formalized application process.

The conundrum in building academic programmes/departments is whether to focus on one or two areas of research, investing in able leaders/researchers and recruiting only those who wish to study alongside them, or alternatively to have a broader base. Larger schools may have this privilege for strategic planning. However, having more areas of research is an attractive proposition if there are several research-able academics/faculty members in the field and it is not vulnerable to the vicissitudes of grant holders. In Brazil, the areas of interest in doctoral programmes are related to different research lines in each programme. The leaders of the nursing area at CAPES/MEC (MEC/CAPES, 2001), jointly with graduate programme coordinators and supervisors, have delineated the most frequently researched lines in the country. These lines include professional, clinical and organizational fields.

According to Carvalho (2002), the professional category must be understood as comprising the sociopolitical space of the profession and includes studies concerning theoretical, philosophical, historical and ethical fundamentals, as well as the technological production in the area. The clinical category refers to the objective reality that can be perceived, thought about and represented. Hence, the care given to human beings during the health and disease process is considered in this category. Finally, the organizational category is related to the nurse's profession in the context of service management, health and education practices, and participation in public policies.

Student quality

Admission criteria, process and issues

Admission procedures are becoming increasingly more formalized in many countries. Generally, applicants' admission requests are reviewed by admission panels/committees/coordinators of each programme to ensure that criteria are met. Admission criteria usually include the grade point average of the Master's degree or equivalent programme, a brief research proposal, curriculum vitae, previous academic training and qualifications, interview, and language proficiency, if relevant. Many schools in the USA also require satisfactory scores on the Graduate Record Examination or standardized tests. Other admission criteria include good academic skills, an ability to tolerate a measure of uncertainty in their proposed study with the ability to adjust ideas and approaches, and of course, a capacity and willingness for sustained application to study.

Graduates in nursing or a relevant first degree, with preferably a Master's degree in nursing or some postgraduate qualification, usually qualify for admission as postgraduate students in the UK. They then may need to go through one or two processes before being registered as a PhD student. For instance, several universities in the UK admit students to a first-year status of postgraduate student or Master in Philosophy to ensure they have sufficient potential and are able to work on their proposed research project satisfactorily. Subsequently, an upgrading to PhD occurs based on a report submitted on progress and plans for the main PhD project – this includes an interview with other academics. Some colleges of nursing in the USA provide options to apply for the PhD degree from the BSN (Bachelor of Nursing Science) or Master's degree programme, when students show exceptional promise and academic excellence. BSN graduates usually take summer externships for clinical experience and take RN (registered nurse) licensure examination while they continue required courses at the graduate level.

The UK has been keen to improve recruitment and quality and there has been stronger quality control for registration of PhD students. Recommendations across disciplines include emphasizing key or transferrable skills rather than technical skills, giving students more authority over their studies, and introducing four-year programmes with more skills training. These are listed by the UK Quality Assurance Agency (1999, p. 10; see also Box 1.1 in Chapter 1), as: the development of a broad understanding of the context in which the research takes place; analytical and research skills, including the understanding of project design and research methodologies, appropriate to the subject and programme of study; general and employment-related skills, including interpersonal and teamwork skills; project management, information retrieval, and database management; written and oral presentation skills; career planning and advice and intellectual property rights management; language support and academic writing skills; training and support for those researchers who may be involved in teaching and demonstrating activities. In this UK document, a framework for assuring academic quality and standards is also usefully provided.

One major issue with admission is that most students in nursing and midwifery are recruited on a part-time basis. This creates challenges that many other disciplines do not have. Apart from the fact that most graduate students also have family responsibilities and are in paid employment, the elongation of the PhD progress is often difficult to manage (Pearson, 1999). So often student quality has less to do with ability and more to do with responsibilities that may not allow sufficient opportunity for concentrated thinking, data collection and writing. However, when motivated and when proposals utilize the work setting or are part of commissioned work, students can achieve success. Yet, more professionally oriented programmes may also allow for work settings and problems to become part of a study, allowing further opportunities to integrate studies with paid employment (Boore, 1996). While the average time-to-graduation ranges from 3.5–4 years for full-time post-Master's students, it usually is twice as long for part-time students.

Another issue is financial support. The magnitude of need varies as a function of the system. All nursing doctoral programmes in Brazil are linked to public universities that do not charge tuition. Doctoral students can also apply to national financial support agencies for grants in order to develop their theses. To that end, they must apply and submit to a selection process that is conducted by the agency annually. On the other hand, doctoral students in the USA pay tuition and fees from their private funds; scholarships, or predoctoral fellowships are available from the federal government (e.g. the National Institutes of Health) on a competitive basis, with the sponsorship of faculty advisers. In the UK, all students must pay tuition fees. Some may be supported by their employers or Department of Health awards.

Monitoring academic progress

Institutions and faculties are expected to establish processes and resources that monitor progress of the PhD students at different levels and time intervals. Pressure by funding bodies to achieve graduation within a specified time has forced many schools to introduce more systematic monitoring processes. There are two main elements to monitoring academic progress. The first focuses on the individual student and their supervisor or supervisory team. Term or annual progress reports of both students and the academic staff/faculty advisers should be submitted to the faculty committee that monitors academic progress, and steps should be taken if progress is unsatisfactory. This may involve additional support for staff/faculty or a change in the supervisory team/dissertation committee or even interruption of studies if personal circumstances of the student are creating a problem.

The second element is evaluation of the student's programme and the staff/faculty contribution. Supervisors hold the key to progress and have an obligation to support students whenever possible, but they also need support to take some uncomfortable decisions. When students cannot progress, this must be confronted, analysed, and reported. Discontinuation may be necessary, but interruption in studies may be also helpful. Teamwork in a panel and the school/faculty committee is essential to support and not personalize such decisions. Universities have two-way obligations also. They need to provide audit processes and ensure that students are given the support and expertise they require. Yet they also need to ensure that completion rates are satisfactory so that funding agencies approve more resources for future students. For this to happen, collaborative mentorship should be in full action, including facilitative strategies and empowerment of faculty and students (Meleis et al, 1994).

Graduation criteria

The award of a doctorate is seen internationally as a demonstration of competence to work effectively and independently within the discipline and making substantial original contribution to nursing's knowledge base. Recently, other abilities have also been added to these criteria, including the capacity to interrogate those performances in a self-critical text. Satisfactory performance in a written preliminary examination/qualifying examination precedes the formation of the dissertation committee. Final theses/dissertations are expected to demonstrate coherence of thought, originality in research ideas and a comprehensive description of the research process. This should include critical literature reviews, demonstrated competence in research methodology and data analysis, and sophisticated analysis of previous evidence to demonstrate how the new findings add to the knowledge.

Several universities request that the thesis document not be permanently bound when submitted for examination. This allows improvements to be made when suggested by examiners, and it is increasingly rare for candidates to have absolutely no changes recommended. The substantial PhD volume of up to 100,000 words represents a major academic achievement; supervisors have the main responsibility to ensure that the style and content are appropriate to doctoral work. Before submission, a review of the final draft by members of the panel/committee and another peer may help towards high success rates in the process.

Examination of the thesis and taught components is necessarily impartial and essentially involves at least one external academic staff/faculty, who is experienced in supervision and is appointed by a university panel of experts in the field. This *viva voce*, variously conducted as either an interview or public defence of the study, is conducted by the examiners (usually two in the UK and five in Brazil and the USA), who confirm the candidate's depth of knowledge and total involvement in the work as their own contribution (UK Council for Graduate Education, 2002).

Inclusion of published papers as part of the thesis/dissertation is increasingly widespread. This is well established in Scandinavia, where the core of the final thesis has been seen as a logical way to present a programme of work. However, other institutions have favoured a much smaller proportion of the final thesis or report to be presented as papers, considering that the final arbiter of standards should be the examiners rather than editors of the journals. Successful students usually demonstrate scientific production disseminated in scientific meetings and indexed scientific journals, grants, prizes/awards received, a pattern of productive scholarship, and collaboration with researchers in nursing and other disciplines in scientific endeavours.

Resources and infrastructure of the university and school of nursing

Resources

Institutions should have sufficient human, financial, and institutional resources available for research to accomplish the goals of the schools of nursing for doctoral education and faculty research. Because doctoral students work relatively independently, it is essential that they have added academic support and physical resources to exploit. University libraries with information technology experts/advisers are essential for carrying out adequate literature searches and for quiet spaces in which to study. Online facilities should be available wherever students conduct their work. In Brazil, one of the accreditation and re-accreditation criteria of CAPES/MEC is the requirement concerning university infrastructure/resources. The library must have bibliographic collections comprising books, national and international journals in areas that are relevant to the programme's research lines, as well as volumes of dissertations and theses and specific materials such as films and CD-Roms. The libraries must also offer online catalogues, Internet access, CD-Rom databases, and multimedia and study facilities. As a result of technological innovation, various information networks are available for doctoral students, including CAPES' own website (http://www.capes.gov.br), where a variety of journals can be found indexed in the Journal Citation Report (JRC) database and Online Scientific Electronic Library (SCIELO; http://www.scielo.org). This is also where the students have free access to full texts, in addition to library periodicals to facilitate research development. Other sectors, such as audiovisual and scientific documentation facilities, memory centers in Brazil, and others, also provide support to doctoral students (Rodrigues et al, 2002).

Provision of postgraduate facilities is increasingly expected by students, many of whom make heavy personal sacrifices to enrol. Universities should provide space and resources for students; many well-established postgraduate schools have private study areas and social areas with dedicated staff who are responsive and on hand to provide advice to students.

Infrastructure

Administrative support should always be clearly identified with every school/faculty. Availability of personnel is essential for doctoral students who have queries regarding procedures, payment of fees, registration, or submission. Information handbooks are essential as well; hard copies and web-based versions should be issued annually. Administrators who are knowledgeable and helpful can make a real difference to the success of a programme. They can produce promotional materials, arrange open days, create a good network among students and provide all necessary web-based information that is readily available. They also service the doctoral committees, keep supervisors aware of their duties, and maintain all the necessary databases. In addition, personal tutors may also help in the (hopefully exceptional) occasions when the supervisory relationship is problematic, by representing students' problems to staff panels.

An essential feature of doctoral support is appeals procedures. In the unfortunate eventuality of failure and dispute over examiners' judgement, students need to be clear that there is a higher or alternative route by which they can be re-examined. This should not be cumbersome, too time-consuming, or embarrassing for examiners. Audit of the frequency, outcome and cost of appeals should be fully documented and maintained by university administrators.

Research-intensive institutions usually have an office of research administration that keeps a record of peer-reviewed external funding, postdoctoral programmes, and internal research funds, as well as providing grant management services. In the USA, 56 schools (86.2%) had designated research support offices (Yoon et al, 2002). In addition, many nursing schools of exceptional quality have centres of research excellence and endowed professorships.

Quality monitoring and evaluation of doctoral programmes

Quality monitoring

In Brazil, the existence of a teaching and research base is the key component in the evaluation of the quality of doctoral education (Guimaraes, 1996). Research groups in doctoral programmes are registered in the Directory of Doctoral Programmes Research Groups of the National Council for Scientific and Technological Development (CNPQ)/Ministry of Science and Technology (http://www.cnpq.br) available to the scientific community. The participation of doctoral students in these groups has favoured greater development in research and, as a result, its dissemination in scientific meetings and periodicals. In addition to research results, the theoretical experience of the doctoral students has shown noticeable differences in the work market, particularly for academicians. According to the evaluation by undergraduates, graduates and supervisors, faculty qualification has allowed doctoral students to have closer contact with academic reality. The tripod of education, science and technology constitutes the base for the progress of graduate programmes in Brazil.

The success of doctoral work across a faculty may be evaluated by the number of successful graduates from each cohort who complete their doctorate within the recommended timescale. However, their experience and relationship with academic staff/faculty is equally important, given that one reason for training doctoral students is to produce the next generation of academic scholars. Important research is undertaken as part of doctoral programmes, and staff should invest energy in helping students. Staff too, gain from the process as their curriculum vitae cite the number of successful candidates they have supervised and joint papers they have published.

Faculty should have earned a doctoral degree with a programme of research that is externally funded and have ongoing peer-reviewed publications of research, theory, ethical or philosophical essays. They should also be involved in scientific review activities of government funding agencies such as the National Institutes of Health study sections in the USA, and other grant application review groups and/or editorial review activities. They should have national or international recognition as scholars in an identified area and demonstrate evidence of influence on science policy throughout the field. Faculty should devote a significant proportion of time to dissertation advisement; generally, each faculty member should serve as the major adviser/chair for no more than three to five students during the dissertation phase.

In nursing, students often choose to work with a specific member of staff/faculty because of their expertise, personality and previous success rate with doctoral candidates. Increasing specialization of postgraduate tutors/faculty members may mean that six to eight students, whether full or part time, can be appropriately supervised by one faculty during the programme of study.

Established doctoral schools tend to be epitomized by clearly documented regulations, procedures for audit and evaluation, dedicated faculty, and a cohort of students who have regular seminars, good representation, and easy access to staff. In time, academics have learned that they too flourish through creating a group of well-prepared doctoral students who, after graduation, may rapidly overtake them in research ideas and productivity.

Increasingly, the quality of doctoral education is judged by the achievements of alumni in society and the number of postdoctoral fellows in the nursing unit (college or department). Their contributions as leaders or leading members of policy-making bodies, corporate and academic institutions, clinical practice settings and social welfare agencies, both nationally and internationally, are credible proxy measures of quality outcomes of doctoral education. The degree to which the institution carries the training programme for postdoctoral fellows is another indicator of the maturity of the faculty research activities; hence, it is an excellent measure of the quality outcome of the doctoral education.

Quality monitoring of doctoral programmes varies widely among countries, ranging from a highly centralized government approach to a decentralized one in which individual universities bear the major responsibility of self-monitoring with periodic regional accreditation systems. Brazil belongs to the first category and the USA to the latter.

Quality evaluation

In Brazil, the Evaluation Board of the CAPES/MEC evaluates national graduate programmes (new programmes and those in progress) and coordinates the work performed by the consultants who analyse the merit of applications for grants abroad, support linked to CAPES' sponsoring programmes and dissemination of the statistical data concerning graduate programmes (MEC/CAPES, 2002). The evaluation is done using a scale with scores from 1 to 7, the latter being the maximum score for doctoral programmes. For instance, scores 6 and 7 are only awarded to programmes offering excellent doctorates according to international standards for the area. Doctoral programmes present annual follow-up reports that include continuing evaluation; however, the final evaluation is conducted triennially (e.g. 2001, 2002 and 2003 at once). This process has been constructed with the participation of the scientific community and has been conducted by academic peers. Nursing has been placed in the larger health science areas, whose criteria are homogenous and respect the particularities of that field of knowledge. This inclusion enables greater visibility of nursing, as it is given the same scientific status as other knowledge areas.

Brazil has a national evaluation system for graduate programmes. Article I of the Resolution by the Federal Education Council (CNE) expresses that, *stricto sensu*, graduate programmes, including doctorates, are subject to requirements such as programme authorization, accreditation and accreditation renewal. Authorization applies only to having the project approved by CNE based on evaluations conducted by CAPES. Hence, all doctoral programmes must begin their activities only after their approval by CAPES/MEC.

With the new evaluation model for Brazilian graduate programmes, there has been a progressive consolidation of programmes. However, many items must still be discussed and implemented. The nursing evaluation committee (1998–2000) mentions that interlocution among area representatives and committees has been intensified; nevertheless, it reports that, many times, changing the evaluation criteria in a short period of time damages the area (Erdmann et al, 2002). By taking into account that international scientific production is a strong quality indicator of doctoral programmes, nursing is re-discussing its inclusion in international events, projects, and exchange programmes, in addition to 'sandwich doctorates' (training in international universities during the doctoral programme) and at the postdoctorate level for greater scientific productivity, which allows for greater international visibility of the Brazilian scientific production.

In the USA, the evaluation plan included in the Position Statement of the American Association of Colleges of Nursing (2001) serves as a useful guide. In many ways, AACN has been the watchdog for the quality of doctoral programmes, but it does not have the formal authority to judge the quality of programmes. AACN holds an annual conference on doctoral education in which most doctoral programme directors and deans of the colleges of nursing participate and discuss various aspects of doctoral education. It has published a set of indicators for quality doctoral education since 1986; the latest revision was published in November 2001, *Indicators of Quality in Research-Focused Doctoral Programs in Nursing*. This document addresses overall indicators of quality for each domain of concern (criteria), but standards *per se* are not included. AACN noted that the ideal evaluation plan is:

> systematic, ongoing, comprehensive, and focuses on the university's and program's specific mission and goals; includes both process and outcome data related to these indicators of quality in research-focused doctoral programs; adheres to established ethical and process standards for formal program evaluation, involves students and graduates in evaluation activities; includes data from a variety of internal and external constituencies;

> provides for comparison of program processes and outcomes to the standards of its parent graduate school/university and selected peer groups within nursing; includes ongoing feedback to program faculty, administrators and external constituents to promote program improvement; and provides comprehensive data to determine patterns and trends and recommend future directions at regular intervals; and is supported with adequate human, financial, and institutional resources.
>
> (AACN, 2001, p. 6)

These principles are echoed by the Quality Assurance Agency of the UK. In addition, examples of a similar programme evaluation for a professional doctorate have been provided by Ingleton et al (2001) and Germain et al (1994).

In the USA, the universities and their respective boards of trustees, and the state boards of higher education approve the doctoral programmes. Once approved, the universities receive accreditation by the regional accreditation authorities of higher education on a regular basis. Quality monitoring of doctoral programmes in nursing in the USA is largely self-directed by the colleges of nursing with oversight of the graduate school, if the university has one. National accreditation by either the National League for Nursing or the Commission on Collegiate Nursing Education is for the baccalaureate and Master's programmes, and doctoral programmes are not official components of these specialized accreditation systems.

Feedback from students is now documented annually in most schools/faculties and shared at the university/college level. A recent internal report of the colleges of the University of London found valuable feedback from their students regarding their experience. Seventy-five per cent had a warm relationship with their supervisors; 70% wanted academic freedom, and for most this exists; and all students wanted more administrative structure in their relationship with their supervisors. Staff may not wholly accept sanctions for poor supervising, but students should be able to change supervisors in any event. Staff can be re-trained or return to co-supervision if they constantly receive poor feedback.

Most universities aim to increase the population of doctoral students to as much as 30% of the total student population, recognizing their worth for future research and academic life. In the UK, this is happening rapidly, and the associated emphasis on quality assurance has influenced further investment and energy by administrative and academic staff. Aiming at a substantial research-active community in the UK, nursing is only realistic if doctoral preparation is excellent. Needless to say, having a critical mass of active researchers in the schools of nursing will ensure the quality of the doctoral programme, thus contributing to excellence in evaluation.

Global quality criteria: work of the INDEN QCI

To address the issue of quality of doctoral education in nursing at the global level, the International Network for Doctoral Education in Nursing (INDEN) launched a committee on quality criteria, standards and indicators (QCI). A 16-member committee from eight countries has worked collaboratively on this project for more than two years, and the eighth draft was distributed to all INDEN members for their review and input in 2002. The eight countries represented by the committee members are Australia, Brazil, Canada, Korea, Poland, South Africa, the UK and the USA. This document focused on one type of doctoral programme, namely on research-intensive programmes (following the AACN definition) regardless of the title (e.g. PhD, DNS, D. Curatonis) awarded upon graduation. This would include programmes that require coursework as well as research-only programmes with little or no coursework. The latter approach is common in Europe, Australia and several other countries, where an apprenticeship relationship between the student and the major adviser constitutes the mainstay of the programme. It should be noted that the aforementioned AACN Position Statement (2001) played a major role in formulating the quality criteria and indicators. Limitations of space preclude the inclusion of its content here. INDEN expects to publish its document in the near future. This chapter has provided in-depth information about the three countries the authors represent.

Conclusions

The authors are pleased to note that we all agree about the importance of quality monitoring for doctoral education in nursing, particularly in the light of the rapid growth of its programmes across countries. However, we observe that a shortage of qualified faculty poses a serious threat to the quality of doctoral education in most countries. Educating and training doctoral students from a younger age is one solution we must pursue seriously. Our collaborative efforts revealed that there are more similarities than differences concerning issues related to components, monitoring methods and evaluation procedures of the quality of doctoral programmes in nursing among the three countries we represent. The same can be said about the approaches each country takes to address these issues. However, the processes for achieving the same goal of quality are different, as education systems are different in the three countries.

To improve the overall quality of doctoral education in nursing, we see a need for developing global quality criteria, standards and indicators. To this end, the work of the QCI committee of the INDEN holds promise. Last but not least, we must strengthen faculty research portfolios, improve resources and infrastructure for effective operations of doctoral programmes, and increase funding for research and scholarly activities of faculty and students.

The criteria, standards and indicators described in this chapter are expected to be applicable in varying degrees to different types of doctoral degrees and different modes/approaches to doctoral education. However, concern might be raised about curriculum/programme evaluation criteria for programmes where the primary mode of study is through research with a primary mentor, with no formal coursework. In response, we would note that student progress in research must be monitored with care over time to determine whether satisfactory progress is occurring. Standards have to be set, with specific indicators determined to measure the degree of progress in the particular areas of study the student is focusing on.

Similarly, concern has been raised about whether criteria/standards/indicators regarding students are applicable in instances where the student will be pursuing research through one-to-one supervision with a mentor. The answer is a resounding yes. The quality of admitted students is an important determinant of the quality of graduates, and the type of roles they will assume upon graduation, and hence, of programme quality. Regardless of the type of programme students are enrolled in, they need to be mentored to undertake gradually more rigorous and demanding scholarly tasks, prepare proposals and compete with peers, and demonstrate success in obtaining funding for research and for projects involving innovative educational and service initiatives.

We acknowledge that while not all the criteria may be applicable to all types of programmes, the described criteria are sufficiently flexible to be adapted to specific circumstances, and used to guide educational activities.

References

American Association of Colleges of Nursing (2001). *Indicators of quality in research-focused doctoral programs in nursing*. Washington, DC: AACN (http://www.aacn.nche.edu (accessed on 9.03.2004)).

Anderson, C. A. (2000). Current strengths and limitations of doctoral education in nursing: Are we prepared for the future? *Journal of Professional Nursing*, **16**(4), 191–200.

Boore, J. R. P. (1996). Doctoral level education in the health professions. *Teaching in Higher Education*, **1**(1), 29–47.

Carvalho, V. (2002). Nursing research lines and priorities – proposal with gnoseologic distinction for the grouping of post-graduate scientific production in nursing. *Rev Esc Anna Nery*, **6**(1), 145–54.

Erdmann, A. L., Leite, J. L., Pagliuca, L. M. F., Almeida, M. C. P., Gutierrez, M. G. R., and Kurcgant, P. (2002). *Nursing Evaluation. Infocapes, Brasília*, **10**(3), 56–60.

Germain, C. P., Deatrick, J. A., Hagopian, G. A., and Whitney F. W. (1994). Evaluation of PhD program: Paving the ways. *Nursing Outlook*, **42**(3), 117–122.

Guimaraes, R. (1996). Post graduation and research. In: *Ministério da Educação e do Desporto*. [Discussion about Brazil post graduation]. Vol 1. Brasilia: CAPES, pp. 9–18.

Ingleton, C., Ramcharan, P., Ellis, L. and Schofield, P. (2001). Introducing a professional doctorate in nursing and midwifery. *Bristol Journal of Nursing*, **1**(22), 1489–1476.

Lash, A. (1992). Determinants of career attainments of doctorates in nursing. *Nursing Research*, **41**(4), 216–222.

MEC/CAPES. CAPES, Brazil. (2002). *Action lines and programs–2003.CAPES*, Brazil.

Meleis, A., Hall, J. and Stevens, P. (1994). Scholarly caring in doctoral nursing education: Promoting diversity and collaborative mentorship. *Image – Journal of Nursing Scholarship,* **26**(3), 177–180.

Minnick, A. and Halstead, L. (2002). A data-based agenda for doctoral nursing education reform. *Nursing Outlook,* **50**(1), 24–29.

Pearson, M. (1996). Professional PhD evaluation to enhance the quality of the student experience. *Higher Education,* **32**, 303–320.

Pearson, M. (1999). The changing environment for doctoral education in Australia: implications for quality management, improvement and innovation. *Higher Education Research and Development,* **18**(3), 269–287.

Quality Assurance Agency for Higher Education (1999). *Code of practice for the assurance of academic quality and standard in higher education, post-graduate research programme.* Gloucester: QAA.

Rodrigues, R. A. P., Erdmann, A. L., Silva, I. A., Fernandes, J. D., Santos, R. S., & Araújo, T. L. (2002). The formation of PhDs in nursing in Brazil. *Texto & Contexto Enfermagem, Florianópolis,* **11**(02), 66–76.

Schmitt, M. H. (1999). Going international in doctoral education in nursing: The creation of INDEN [Editorial]. *Research in Nursing and Health,* **22**, 355–356.

UK Council for Graduate Education (2002). *Professional doctorates.* (http://www.ukcge.ac.uk (accessed on 9.07.2004)).

Yoon, S., Wolfe, S., Yucha, C. and Tsai, P. (2002). Research support by doctoral-granting colleges/schools of nursing. *Journal of Professional Nursing,* **18**(1), 16–21.

Chapter 10

Emergent forms of doctoral education in nursing

Mary Courtney, Kate Galvin, Carla Patterson and Lillie M. Shortridge-Baggett

This chapter provides an overview of the differentiation between the 'non-taught' and 'taught' doctorates, and examines why and how different doctoral approaches in nursing have evolved. The major forms of doctoral education examined are: professional doctoral programmes (mainly taught), doctorates by published work, and doctorates by portfolio; doctoral study via distance education is also explored. Within our discussion we draw out benefits and challenges of these diverse doctoral approaches in nursing, all of which are equally robust and aim to contribute to knowledge for practice.

For the purpose of the chapter doctorates may be termed 'non-traditional doctorates'; however, we acknowledge that it is difficult to define what is traditional and non-traditional[1] in a global context. We suggest that because many different doctoral education systems have emerged over time in many countries with distinct postgraduate systems, no single definition is satisfactory, and mutually exclusive criteria to categorize doctorates are difficult to identify. While many countries have examples of 'traditional' PhDs by thesis, diverse new approaches to doctoral education are emerging worldwide, some based on the US Doctorate of Nursing Science (DNS) model, with others emerging within specific contexts such as practice and/or higher education policy, and are subsequently mixed in their structure and delivery.

Therefore, we explore new forms of doctoral education as well as concepts that underpin current understandings of the non-taught (thesis-based PhD) and taught doctorates (professional doctorates such as DNS), and illustrate their key tenets.

Taught and non-taught doctorates

The development of doctorates in nursing has given rise to two different doctoral systems: the taught (professional doctorate such as the DNS) and the non-taught (PhD degree by research thesis). A general differentiation can be made between traditional European-style PhD and taught professional doctorate routes; a PhD is an academic or research degree, whereas a DNS or its equivalent title is a clinical and *application of research* degree. Several published papers support such a differentiation and indicate a need for diverse routes (Seitz, 1987; Blancett, 1989; McKenna and Cutcliffe, 2001), with varied purpose.

The PhD is a research-orientated degree to train students for scholarly or research activities. It is directed towards generation of new knowledge and requires at least three years of full-time study where capacity for original research and new contribution to knowledge must be demonstrated (UK Council for Graduate Education [UKCGE], 2002). In those countries offering PhD by thesis formal guidance and structure are provided via a supervisory process. Commonly, the student's PhD research proposal will be formally peer reviewed by the school or faculty research committee, which will appoint a supervisor(s) with appropriate expertise. Because the PhD is attained via a successful 80,000–100,000-word thesis only, historically it has not been a requirement that students attend lectures or undertake examinations or coursework. Increasingly, however, PhD students are encouraged to undertake research methodology training and more universities are establishing research graduate schools where students will be supported with formal research training (Higher Education Funding Council of England, 2002).

Within a typical supervisory process the supervisor(s) and student will explore the aims and objectives, methodological approach, and feasibility of the study, sample availability and whether ethical approval will be possible. The supervisor(s) will also oversee data collection and write-up. The process culminates in an oral examination of the thesis by an external examiner who is an expert in the field or a panel. In Australia, in the majority of universities, the examination process is undertaken by forwarding the completed thesis to two to three external independent examiners who forward their written decision to the university.

In contrast, the taught doctorate, or professional doctorate (DNS), is a practice-orientated professional degree to prepare students for higher level professional practice and leadership. Usually, three years of full-time study are required (although part-time equivalents are emerging in some countries), which is directed towards transmission and application of existing knowledge, to strengthen the evidence base of nursing with the focus of research being the solution of problems in practice and the generation of new knowledge to inform improvement in practice.

Reason for the evolution of different doctorates

Established taught nursing doctorates have developed rapidly over a long period in the USA. A modular system of doctoral education emerged in the 1920s. The first programme was established at Columbia University, in 1924 – a Doctorate of Education. The first nursing doctorate, DNS, emerged in the 1960s (Flaherty, 1989; Ketefian et al, 2001). Subsequently, other US universities introduced other variations, such as the Doctorate of Nursing Science (DNSc), Doctorate of Nursing (DNurs or DN), and Doctorate of Science in

Nursing (DSN) (Pearson et al, 1997). Anderson (2000) reports incremental development of doctoral programmes since their inception: 1954, n = 2; 1977, n = 17; 1985, n = 29; 1990, n = 50; 1999, n = 70. Murphy (1981) describes distinct phases, arguing that initially programmes educated nurses for functional roles, whereas, from the 1970s, the shift was towards education about nursing. Ketefian et al (2001) have recently reported that the USA offers nursing doctorates from over 85 institutions. They highlight variations in style of delivery and titles but conclude that the majority of programmes have a period of taught coursework followed by engagement in one or more research projects and a final dissertation. These taught doctorates require similar amounts of credit, and present a similar modularized form covering most commonly research methods, theory development, specialization in an area of nursing science, teaching, leadership and dissertation (International Network for Doctoral Education in Nursing, 2002). In contrast, Australia has followed the traditional PhD approach, having a strong history of non-taught doctorates (PhD by research thesis) with taught doctorates having a slow uptake. In 2003, of the 37 Australian universities offering nursing education, only five offered a professional doctorate in nursing with varying forms of nomenclature used, e.g. Doctor of Nursing Science and Doctor of Health Science with a major in Nursing. There are, however, a number of other professional doctorates in Australia, such as health services management, where the majority of candidates are from the nursing profession and the research undertaken relates directly to nursing practice.

Direct entry into a PhD is generally contingent upon students having previously completed a thesis or dissertation in their Master's degree. The majority of students choosing taught doctorates in Australia tend to do so because direct entry is available without having previously undertaken a Master's thesis. Recent trends demonstrate that more and more Australian Master's level students are choosing to undertake full coursework Master's degrees rather than incorporating the thesis option in their studies, and therefore it is envisaged that future demand for 'taught doctorates' in Australia will increase in years to come.

The UK experience, like Australia, saw the development of professional doctorate education much later (60 years) than the North American developments. Bourner et al (2001) report that while these new approaches to doctoral education have been relatively slow to develop in the UK, there has been exponential growth in the past five years, the major drivers being the increased vocational focus of universities and problems with PhDs in practice disciplines (Galvin and Carr, 2003). Traditional PhD programmes have been criticized in the UK, with evidence that they do not always meet the needs of the industry in providing competent postdoctoral researchers, and have also been criticized as being too narrow (Booth, 2001). For example, Traynor and Rafferty (1998) estimate that there were 283 completed nursing PhDs in the years between 1976 and 1993. A number of issues were identified concerning the output of these traditional doctorates: a clinical practice focus with the potential for direct impact on patient care was weak, with the commonest research questions concerning professional issues such as workforce characteristics, service organization, management and industrial relations. As expected, the most established UK universities produced the highest number of PhDs. Traynor and Rafferty's study provides evidence of the need for further innovation to ensure both discipline development and future impact on clinical practice as a result of doctoral level work.

The first Doctorate in Nursing Science in Europe was established at the University of Ulster in 1995 (Boore, 1997). Boore (1996) describes the curriculum which leads to a Doctorate in Nursing Science (DNS), which is modular in structure and covers three main but integrated areas: theory development, acquisition of specialist knowledge and research. She argues that graduates (doctors of nursing science) will 'have the knowledge base to be able to function at an advanced level and to be able to function and to develop into expert clinical practitioners, advisors, managers or educators within their particular area of expertise' (Boore, 1996, p. 623). By 2003, there were six new providers of 'taught' doctorates in nursing in the UK and further programmes are in development.

Interestingly, there has been a long and ongoing debate about the purpose and nature of PhDs in social sciences compared with PhDs in the natural sciences (Advisory Board for the Research Councils, 1993), which reflects some of the discipline-based debates; for instance, Boore (1996) indicates that within science the approach was generally to provide 'training', while within social sciences the emphasis has been 'the knowledge PhD'.

In nursing and midwifery, additional difficulties with the non-taught PhD have also been identified, such as inadequate funding for full-time study; a lack of 'structure'; problems with the application of traditional research processes in practice disciplines, and problems with regard to part-time study, which does not always strengthen research and practice links sufficiently (Mason and McKenna, 1995). The PhD by research thesis has been described as a long and lonely endeavour with high rates of non-completion; it is of note that many nurses are also in high-pressure clinical roles and are not funded (Galvin and Carr, 2003). The average age of PhD students in nursing is 35 years compared with 25 years in the basic sciences; most students study part time after several years in clinical practice rather than studying full time directly after completion of an undergraduate degree as is the case in the basic sciences (McKenna and Cutcliffe, 2001). Therefore, the taught doctorate is attractive to students who may enjoy peer group support and coursework milestones. Additionally, some programmes are supported by a 'graduate school' structure (shared learning with other professionals via graduate school seminars with other disciplines). Most professional doctorates in UK nursing departments have 'nursing' in the title of the award, and although focused on nursing, some share units and therefore share teaching with other professionals. Clinical nursing might be the focus; however, interdisciplinary learning is also an important feature for some.

Evolution and nature of doctoral programmes

Professional doctorates are not new and have emerged in a wide range of disciplines; for example, Doctor of Education (DEd); Doctor of Psychology (DPsych); Doctor of Dental Science (DDS); Doctor of Physical Therapy (DPT). By tracing their historical roots, their purpose can be explored. The range of doctorates in a multiprofessional context has been outlined with a short description of their history by Pierce and Peyton (1999). Several professional doctorates, including DDS and Doctor of Pharmacy (PharmD) have reflected the historical roots of the Doctor of Medicine (MD) degree. The MD has a long history; at its inception in the USA the MD was a baccalaureate degree with acquisition of clinical skills based on an apprenticeship model. Pierce and Peyton (1999) argue that these three degrees were driven by a requirement to enhance practitioners' competence in clinical practice.

> The success of these three fields in their adoption of similar curricular models emphasising a preliminary degree, advanced education, higher standards for entry, research-based practice and extended clinical internships recommends this approach to practitioner education as one that has proven effective.
>
> (Pierce and Peyton, 1999, p. 66).

Within nursing, an early definition of a professional doctorate in nursing provided by Newman (1975) reflects historical parallels with MD degrees:

> A *professional* doctorate is not to be confused with an *academic* doctorate. The latter, the PhD, is an advanced research degree, preceded by basic undergraduate education in the field and is intended to prepare scholars who will advance and teach knowledge in the field. In contrast, a professional doctorate is a practice degree similar to the doctor of medicine degree and constitutes basic preparation for practice.
>
> (Newman, 1975, p. 705).

Note that Newman was discussing an ND degree (Nursing Doctorate), conceived as the entry level practice degree, similar to the MD, DDS and PharmD. This degree is currently offered by three institutions within the USA.

As already described, provision of doctorates in nursing has developed within different international postgraduate arenas with different histories and structures. Historically, the main drivers for US doctorates were to prepare 'faculty'. Murphy's analysis (1981) concludes that from 1926 to 1959 a generation of nurses who undertook educational doctorates were prepared for functional roles mainly in teaching settings, whom she labels 'the functional specialists'. Later, doctorates placed emphasis upon nursing theory and clinical issues which reflected both developments in healthcare in that decade and the disciplinary focus of nursing (1960–1969) – the 'nurse scientists'. Finally, a cadre of nurse scholars emerged whose doctorates *of* nursing were focused on knowledge development *in* nursing (from the 1970s).

A major influence has been the increasing specialization in clinical practice as evidenced by a growing provision of clinically specialized Master's courses (Cotton, 1997), and increased clinical specialization within doctoral programmes (Bigbee, 1996). Therefore, doctorates have changed in both structure and focus over time, reflecting an increased demand for specialist roles in education, clinical practice and management, at both preregistration and postgraduate levels.

Other US literature has also emerged which describes new types of doctorates labelled 'non-traditional' (Pickard, 1986; Scott and Conrad, 1992; Sakalys et al, 1995). These authors describe programmes that are intensive and concentrated in shorter time spans (for example 'over the Summer' such as that provided by University of Colorado Health Sciences Center). These are programmes that meet both a professional and an adult learning agenda and are a direct response to the high demand for doctorally prepared clinicians, who find the typical programme inflexible, or not provided locally. These 'non-traditional' programmes have an overall goal of facilitating adult learners to develop professionally at the same time as overcoming problems related to full-time study and geographical inaccessibility, perhaps ideally suited to both clinicians and managers. In 1995, six US universities offered intensive summer-only options and demand was reported as very high (Sakalys et al, 1995). Evaluation of the programmes suggest that they are commensurate in quality and levels of student satisfaction but that they have a potential to cause stress and fatigue (Scott and Conrad, 1992; Sakalys et al, 1995).

Elsewhere, doctorates for specific professionals have been slower to emerge (Bourner et al, 2001), and the earliest programmes were made available in 1992 (the Doctorate of Education at Bristol University). Prolific development followed, and by 1998 there were 109 programmes available in 19 subjects. Bourner et al report that medicine, business administration, education, psychology and engineering account for almost 80% of the programmes, but that there is a growing range of subjects. In addition, part-time study programmes have increased in number, reflecting the increasing demand for postgraduate study with professional and personal development aims (UKCGE, 2002). The disciplines relevant to health and social care and the number of programmes that were in existence in 1998 are summarized as follows: Doctor of Education, 29; Doctor of Medicine, 20; Doctor of Clinical Psychology, 19; Doctor of Business Administration, 9; Doctor of Psychology, 4; Doctor of Educational Psychology, 4; Doctor of Public Health, 1; Doctor of Occupational Psychology, 1; Doctor of Clinical Science, 1 (Bourner et al, 2001).

It is of note that a number of doctorates in business administration have also evolved, perhaps reflecting increasing demand for professional practice and personal development in the business and industry sector. These too may be attractive to managers in the healthcare sector (Holloway and Walker, 2000). There are also a large number of educational doctorates often attractive to nurse educationalists. In summary, a range of doctorates have emerged that are distinct from the traditional PhD, which aim to underpin the needs of specific professional groups relevant to nursing. They reflect a range of learning outcomes specific to professional needs in practice. The UK Council for Graduate Education (2002) defines the nature of these doctorates as:

> a programme of advanced study and research which, whilst satisfying the University criteria for the award of a doctorate, is designed to meet the specific needs of a professional group external to the University, and which develops the capability of individuals to work within a professional context.
>
> (UKCGE, 2002, p. 62)

Galvin and Carr (2003) have reported students' perceptions of the increasing opportunities for nurses to engage in professional doctorates in nursing, with several UK programmes in existence in 2000. Due to the curriculum requirements placed on British universities (Bourner et al, 2001) most share a common structure with a range of 'taught core units of study' and a thesis.

Galvin and Carr (2003) have observed that most nursing doctorates comprise core units, delivered as taught modules or through the seminar approach. A major feature is the requirement of a thesis with reduced length (40,000–60,000 words) compared to the traditional thesis of 80,000–100,000 words. In their study 'New knowledge for improvement' they describe the underlying programme mission from data generated by course leaders about the aims guiding the nursing doctorates.

In a small study of professional doctorate students Galvin and Carr (2002) also highlighted that practice-focused careers rather than academic careers are prominent aspirations; the motivation for doctoral study among their sample was to contribute to practice and have an impact on patient care. However, the findings also showed the need for expertise in a wide range of research methods; they report that a broad skill set within a context of multiprofessional care delivery is not fully acknowledged by existing doctoral students. The features of healthcare practice provide a clear rationale for multiple doctorate programmes that are both traditional and non-traditional and that facilitate clinicians, educators and managers. Most UK doctorates are primarily focused on meeting particular professional needs, often reflected in their titles (e.g. Doctor of Administration, Doctor of Finance, Doctor of Counselling Psychology, Doctor of Nursing Science). However, a small number of universities in the UK offer generic professional doctorate programmes with the content negotiable with the student to meet personal and professional needs (for example, Doctor of Professional Studies or Doctor of Professional Practice). In addition, interprofessional educational strategies are beginning to emerge (UKCGE, 2002).

Challenges and benefits to nursing

A complicating feature of the international literature is that numerous definitions have been used to describe a diversity of courses of study. Within the discipline of nursing, a wide range of offerings, both thesis-based and primarily taught have emerged; some are at the post-registration level, some at the clinical entry, and some at the postgraduate level. In addition, some have a research or practice focus or both (Lancaster, 1984; Ziemer et al, 1992). Furthermore, different aims, patterns of course delivery and philosophy have emerged as doctorates have been developed internationally, confusing the picture further. For example, the US system contrasts sharply, with an absence of professional registration at the doctoral level for nursing, seen in many other countries, where the focus has been on nursing theory and science, research training and professional and educational issues.

The state of development of the literature reflects the concentration of doctorates globally, with many North American, UK and Australian papers. A number of challenges within specific doctoral programmes are apparent; however, less is known about doctoral developments on a truly international scale. Therefore, the existing literature provides some differentiation between traditional PhDs and professional doctorate programmes in some specific countries, but does not clarify the differentiation between diverse doctoral models in a worldwide context.

A few studies have indicated inherent problems in differentiation between the aims and the philosophy of programmes (Lancaster, 1984; Downs, 1989; Hudacek and Carpenter, 1998). Challenges include providing clarity between the aims of professional doctorates and their structure, differentiating their philosophy and the nature of any thesis from that of the PhD by thesis, and being clear about roles they prepare students for. Doncaster and Thorne (2000) provide helpful terminology to differentiate these roles, the 'professional scholar' and the 'scholarly professional'. The non-taught doctorate (by thesis) aims to develop professional scholars who will lead and support academic developments and research, whilst the taught doctorate (professional doctorate) aims to produce scholarly professionals who practise with sophisticated knowledge to inform practice that includes evaluation of evidence and critical reflection.

Against this backdrop, however, all doctoral theses, regardless of the format in which they have been compiled, have common objectives:

- to undertake an original inquiry which makes a substantial contribution to nursing knowledge
- to successfully complete their doctoral studies in their chosen area of research interest
- to provide evidence of the quality of the student's understanding of the work undertaken

- to demonstrate to examiners that the inquiry undertaken has made an appropriate contribution to advancing knowledge.

Doctoral students have a diverse range of opportunities to exploit during doctoral study. Reflection upon the nature of their current role, learning style and future aspirations for career development will determine their choice of programme. In addition, internationally, the diverse range of programmes adds to the rich potential to develop the nursing discipline further in both academic and practice settings.

Three major forms of non-traditional doctoral education will now be examined: doctorates by published work and doctorates by portfolio, followed by a discussion on undertaking doctoral study by distance education.

Doctorates by published work

Traditionally, the doctoral thesis has been written in a monograph format using a series of standard chapter headings such as Introduction, Literature Review, Methodology, Results, Discussion and Conclusion. However, in recent years, an alternative model for writing a thesis has emerged and we see many universities now giving students the option to write their thesis by published work. The thesis by publication approach is a well-established method in certain disciplines and some leading universities worldwide. This approach ensures that the candidate has pursued rigorous research and is recognized as a scholar in the field through ongoing professional activities, grant writing, presentations, as well as submitting refereed articles for publication. These activities are undertaken prior to submitting the final thesis monograph for review and public defence by an expert panel of professors and other scientists. Undertaking the doctorate this way permits the candidate to 'develop an in depth knowledge of the domain of study' and the student becomes very 'self-directed' (Grypdonck, 2001, p. 6).

This approach does not require that compulsory prescribed courses be taken before beginning the research investigations or by the time the work is completed. Rather, the candidate is expected to participate in all kinds of research-related activities, including attending seminars, taking courses and/or participating in training sessions (as needed) to conduct the studies and complete several referred publications which will be included in the thesis document, which is subsequently submitted for examination.

It needs to be noted that in the USA, a number of universities granting the PhD allow students to choose the option of presenting their dissertation (thesis) through a series of published articles. However, their programme of study is the same as those students submitting a traditional dissertation, and the procedures for the oral defence are the same for both options.

Two examples of the process used for preparing the doctorate by publication will be given. One is from the University of Utrecht in the Netherlands and the other from Queensland University of Technology (QUT) in Australia. Utrecht, beginning as a school for English missionaries, was officially proclaimed a university in the year 1636, and is now one of the leading research institutions in the world. The University welcomes outstanding students from around the world to obtain a doctorate at over 52 internationally oriented research schools and institutes (University of Utrecht, 2003, http://www.uu.nl/phd). This process takes about four years to complete for full-time study and six years for part-time study (Grypdonck, 2001).

An overview of the process for obtaining a doctorate by research with publications at the University of Utrecht is presented in Table 10.1. Throughout the entire period of study the candidate participates in ongoing professional activities. These activities are noted in the first column of the table. In the next three columns milestones, steps, and publication outcomes are presented. The overall process includes selecting a supervisor and then working with that supervisor to develop a proposal for the doctoral programme, conducting the investigations, and defending the research. Planning for postdoctoral research is a critical category as well. The steps for each of these categories are noted with the desired publications given in the last column.

Of course, the progression is not always as linear as noted in Table 10.1, but an effort is made to have a plan and adhere to the process as closely as possible. One of the potential pitfalls of the process, according to Grypdonck, is that a student might focus on project requirements and that 'the output becomes more important than discovering and learning, including the joy of scholarship' (2001, p. 6).

Obtaining a doctorate by research with publications enables critical appraisal from blinded journal referees during doctoral studies. This leads to the development of a stronger programme of research and assists in reducing flaws in any aspect of the different investigations. The critique provided when presenting a paper at a conference or submitting a manuscript is a very important element in learning research and developing scholarship and scholarly habits.

General format of PhD thesis by published papers

The thesis by publication may comprise:

- published papers
- manuscripts accepted for publication
- manuscripts submitted for publication, or under review.

The minimum number of papers and/or manuscripts required is three, but may be more depending upon the nature of the research study. At least one paper must be published, accepted, or be undergoing revision following refereeing. This number may vary from university to university depending upon local policy. As many refereed papers have multiple authorships, consideration should be given to the number of papers the PhD candidate is principal author for. In the

Table 10.1 Doctorate by published work

Professional activities undertaken throughout doctoral programme	*Milestones*	*Steps*	*Publication outcomes*
Participate in ongoing professional activities Participate in doctoral research seminars	1 Select research area of interest	Identify investigators with a programme of research in area of interest Meet with investigators(s) Discuss process of working together	Complete publication of previous research, especially if the results indicate need for further research in the selected area
Present work throughout the period of doctoral research	2 Develop proposal for investigations as part of the programme	Work with supervisor to develop proposal for doctoral study Undertake preliminary review of literature	Prepare publication with supervisor related to the importance of the area of research
Attend any courses essential to the conduct of the research Attend scientific conferences and meetings Present research at conferences, especially international ones Serve as a consultant in the areas of expertise, especially internationally Maintain currency in areas of study	3 Conduct investigations	Conduct a state of the science literature review on the topic and methods Obtain funding for research studies if possible Conduct a series of studies, for example, validation of instruments, development and/or testing of intervention Conduct controlled clinical trials	Prepare manuscripts with members of the research team Submit manuscript on the state of the science in the selected area of research *(Publication 1)* Submit manuscripts on each phase of the research results, especially to international referred journals *(Publication 2, 3, 4 etc)* Prepare doctoral research monograph with selected scientific publications included

(*cont.*)

Table 10.1 continued

Professional activities undertaken throughout doctoral programme	*Milestones*	*Steps*	*Publication outcomes*
Participate in professional visits related to research, especially internationally	4 Defend doctoral research	Submit doctoral thesis for internal review Submit doctoral thesis for external review Obtain doctoral degree!!!	Complete publication of all manuscripts in preparation following receipt of reviewers' comments Prepare any further publications related to the research *(Publication 5, etc)*
	5 Plan post-doctoral studies	Select an area for further research based on findings of doctoral research Develop a postdoctoral research programme Seek funding for ongoing research	Finalize publication of doctoral publications Develop plan for future publications

QUT model, the candidate must be principal author of at least two of the three papers and must have the written permission of each of the co-authors.

Normally, the thesis should include the following sections:

- Title page
- Key words
- Abstract
- List of publications and/or manuscripts
- Table of contents
- Statement of original authorship
- Acknowledgements
- Introduction
- Literature review
- Methodology (optional)
- Published papers and submitted manuscripts.
- General discussion and conclusion

(Adapted from QUT *Doctor of Philosophy Regulations Chapter 14: Presentation of PhD Theses by Published Papers,* [2003]).

Examination process of thesis by publication

It is usual that all theses, whether submitted by traditional monograph or submitted by publication, are required to undergo formal external examination. Although candidates may have successfully published several refereed research papers on their findings, this does not render the work exempt from formal examination.

Major challenges in thesis production by publication

While different institutions will naturally have variations on the requirements for thesis production whether by publication or in traditional format, some of the challenges in producing a thesis in such a format need to be considered. Such challenges include the time taken to prepare papers for publication; the time taken to gain acceptance; and again the time for the paper to appear in print. Therefore, it is important to consider the timeline for preparing papers in the early stages of the development of the thesis and to be mindful that the structure of some thesis topics may not lend them easily to a thesis by publication. In some instances results may not become available until late in the programme of study and therefore the topic may not lend itself to writing up publication. In such situations it may be possible to publish the results of the pilot study in terms of its development, validation and reliability. Case study 1 provides a suggested thesis format to overcome some of the challenges mentioned.

Case study 1 Using secondary data analysis in undertaking a thesis by publication

This case study describes a format using secondary data analysis, which has worked extremely efficiently for producing a thesis by publication. Not all research questions can be answered in such a way. However, in this case, a preliminary review of the literature revealed that the research questions being asked were important in terms of providing an increased knowledge base in relation to improving health outcomes in an area where knowledge was scant and what was there was outdated.

Example of the content and process of a specific thesis presented by publication

Component	*Process*	*Outcome*	*Advantage*
1 What can be answered in relation to the questions from secondary data analysis from national datasets which are current and available	From analysis of these questions, three subsets of secondary questions are developed and each of these forms the basis of a publication	Three publications in refereed journals which are linked around the original question	The publication process can begin relatively early in the candidature and the papers are cohesive
2 As the secondary data analysis proceeds, gaps emerge	The team works on developing a smaller study which the candidate undertakes to respond to one of these gaps	Publication of component 2	This publication complements the earlier papers so assists in being able to present a logical thesis

The format for writing up the complete thesis by publication is as described previously:

- comprehensive critical literature review
- methods chapter which provides a rationale and detail of the methods utilized, which are often limited in published papers
- four publications
- final linking chapter which generalizes findings from the specific papers, extracts material from the findings which can be used by researchers, policy makers and practitioners for future initiatives, and provides recommendations for future research as well as indicating limitations to the study.

Advantages of thesis production by publication

There are several advantages in preparing a thesis in a format as outlined in case study 1:

- production of a comprehensive focused thesis which can be produced in a limited time
- experience in at least two areas: (i) development of comprehensive data analysis skills; and (ii) understanding experience of the whole process of a small study
- developing skills in writing refereed published papers
- faster dissemination of research findings as papers are written during the course of study rather than waiting until after graduation
- time is utilized more efficiently as there is no requirement to first write a traditional results chapter in the thesis. The student can immediately write the results via a refereed article and this can then be inserted into the body of the thesis
- validation of findings by blinded peer-reviewed journal referees.

Doctorates by portfolio

As already indicated earlier in the chapter, the professional doctorate has emerged as an alternative to the PhD to provide professionals with leadership and advanced skills to solve problems that are directly pertinent to their professions and practice. The question then arises regarding the most appropriate format to achieve this.

An alternative to the conventional thesis

In some instances the conventional product of a doctoral degree, whether it be a traditional-type thesis or the more recently emerging thesis by publication, will be an appropriate format. Indeed PhD theses in some institutions are now accepted as oral histories, as original composition and a range of other formats. There has, however, been criticism of the limitations of these products with such an academic format for reporting the outcomes of research from the professional doctorate which may be undertaken in a very different format to the regular PhD.

We have seen the emergence of the knowledge economy where economies which are likely to thrive in the twenty-first century are those which produce and utilize new knowledge in a wide range of formats; such knowledge needs to be produced in appropriate formats. In instances where the outcome is to introduce a change in practice at the workplace, a large academic text or indeed a series of papers produced for an academic journal may not be the optimal output to achieve such change. A document which contains a range of outputs albeit produced rigorously in an evidence-based, not merely assertive context, may be more appropriate.

Table 10.2 Description of specific components of the structure of a doctorate by portfolio. The title of the thesis portfolio is 'How can government health research policy facilitate research activity and dissemination in field A?

Description of components in the portfolio	*Format and outcome*
1 Introduction	Brief overview of background to the thesis, the research questions and structure and components of the portfolio
2 Succinct critical literature review	This review analyses theoretical frameworks for development and implementation of policy
3 Scoping review of policy development in 'field A' predominantly from the 'grey' literature	The policy review indicates that in 'field A' there is a fragmented approach to policy development. A specific difficulty with multicentre ethics approval is identified
4 Methods section	Summary methods section for all components
5 Identification of why the current ethics process is a barrier and ways of overcoming these barriers	Findings from interviews with ethics committee members, scan of minutes as well as data from a formal audit of the ethics committee and production of new trial ethics guidelines
6 Overview of current research activity including knowledge of researchers of policy within two research institutions at time 1 and time 2	Report written in government report style for future use by policy makers
7 International comparison health research policy development	Refereed academic publication outlining commonalities and differences
8 Final chapter linking all components	This includes pertinent recommendations

Composition of a doctoral portfolio

While most institutions have extremely detailed guidelines outlining how a PhD thesis may be presented, whether it be as a conventional product or through a series of publications, the guidelines for the product of a professional doctorate tend to fall into two categories. The first of these tends to indicate a product which is exactly the same as a PhD and generally the major difference is a reduction in word length, which usually approximates two-thirds of that for a PhD. A number of institutions outline that a portfolio may be acceptable but few provide details of what this might actually look like. Table 10.2 broadly outlines an example of how a portfolio might be put together which would be acceptable for meeting the requirements of the Doctor of Health Science (the umbrella professional doctorate for nursing candidates) at Queensland University of Technology, Australia. The instructions to students are careful to point out that this format is no less rigorous than PhD requirements; indeed, some of the components of the PhD such as a detailed Methods section and a critical Literature Review are included to ensure that the portfolio can be examined in terms of its contribution to the evidence base in the relevant field of practice.

Other portfolios may look quite different from this but the essential features are inclusion of materials suitable for future use in practice as part of the product *per se* rather than those products being couched in a purely academic context. We do not argue that a conventional thesis cannot be the product of a professional doctorate; rather than trying to squeeze something into a format that it does not fit naturally, we advocate that alternative formats be acceptable.

Challenges in producing a portfolio

It will take time and effort to ensure that both supervisors and equally importantly, examiners, are able to come to terms with an alternative format. The real challenge is to provide communication in a format that is relevant to the area where it is hoped the research will impact. It is vital that rigour is maintained in both the conduct of research and its presentation, regardless of format. The challenge is to disseminate to all the value of such outcomes. The question of whether examiners will accept different formats remains to be determined.

Summary of doctorates

There are four major strands to doctoral education specifically relevant to nursing.

- The thesis-based PhD, which is relevant both to nurses undertaking a role in the academy as well as to nurses leading the evidence-based agenda in practice.
- The diverse professional doctorates in nursing, which are available internationally with their focus on the integration of theory, practice and research and are relevant to clinical practice leaders, and to nurses working in education and management. These include a number of intensive programmes that are US-based and which have been labelled in the literature as 'non-traditional'.
- The professional doctorates in a range of relevant and related subjects which will be of interest to some clinicians, educationalists and managers according to the focus of their professional role.
- The generic professional doctorates, which are of interest to a range of health and social care professions, including nurses working in a wide diversity of roles and which offer an interprofessional focus.

Doctoral study by distance education

Increasingly, universities are offering doctoral students the opportunity to undertake their programme of study by distance education (or in the external mode) as opposed to the internal on-campus mode. This initiative is generally in response to prospective students wishing to complete the major component of their PhD candidature at home rather than being located on campus. At Queensland University of Technology, a hybrid of internal and external modes called the 'multi-mode' is offered where students can come to campus for periods of internal study (e.g. two to three months) and then spend the remainder of the year studying externally (by distance education). For example, a student may commence an advanced quantitative research methods unit for the first eight weeks of the semester and then go home and complete the course by distance education. Research supervision contact is maintained via email and fax when the student is off campus.

Benefits for international students

- Cross-cultural understanding for nurses is greatly enhanced when international students are able to undertake their doctoral studies in another country.
- The multi-modal external PhD programme for international students can be individualized to allow students to undertake their studies using a mix of external and internal study at a time which suits their needs.
- Students are able to balance their study commitments with their busy work and family commitments.
- Students can maintain their seniority in employment by not having to resign from their places of employment in order to pursue their studies overseas.
- Gaining access to nursing doctoral studies via distance education makes doctoral study available to students in countries where such nursing studies may not yet be available locally.

Challenges for international students

1. Although university regulations may require students to spend a minimum period on campus, local regulations in the home country may require students to spend at least 12 months overseas during their PhD studies. This results in students spending periods of three months or more per year for four years away from their families and friends to pursue their studies and can result in loneliness while away from home.
2. Achieving English language competency required for entry can be a challenge. Most English language universities require a reasonable level of competence prior to admission to doctoral study. Where the required levels are

not reached, English for Academic Purposes courses are available, as are general English courses. However, again this extends the time that students are away from their homes.

3 Funding for airfares, accommodation and sustenance can be a major challenge for students. Although students who are lecturers are able to come to campus during their student semester breaks and continue to receive their salaries from their home organizations, in many cases they may not receive any funding to support their studies.
4 In many cases, students undertake data collection within their own countries and this can require extensive external supervision. Arrangements are required to engage an external associate supervisor for each multi-modal student to ensure that local supervision is available to assist with gaining access to facilities, ethics approval and advice on data analysis.
5 The student must provide evidence on enrolment that arrangements for the research at the external location (normally a recognized research establishment or place of professional employment) meet the normal requirements of the PhD programme.

Conclusions

It is apparent that doctoral provision in nursing is a rapidly developing area which continues to give rise to a diverse range of non-traditional doctoral education models which exist globally. To a large extent whether or not a doctorate is considered traditional or otherwise is dependent upon higher education and practice context and the inherent history and evolution of postgraduate provision in different parts of the world. As more diverse forms of doctorates emerge, it will be increasingly difficult to define doctorates in terms of taught or non-taught, thesis-based or non-traditional. However, the 'gold standard' of systematic study culminating in original contributions to knowledge remains an important feature for defining 'doctoral level' study. There is an emerging theme within the literature and in the analysis of diverse doctoral programmes which sheds new light on the purpose of the doctorate. We suggest that the models we have described, in addition to further new models, are required to underpin new roles in nursing which are beyond the academic and practice-based research roles. Many postdoctoral nurses may undertake leadership roles in clinical arenas and at policy level, which will require diverse doctoral provision, which is different from a purely 'research training' focus. By commencing the discussion on the differences between non-taught and taught doctorates, and subsequently examining alternative formats to doctoral thesis and assessment we have endeavoured to illustrate the potential benefits and possibilities inherent in varied doctoral education. Additionally, these new and different educational approaches offer much potential to increase doctoral provision globally and to underpin varied nursing roles at postdoctoral level.

Note

1 For example, the 'traditional' doctorate in many European countries and Australasia is thesis-based and different from the 'traditional' DNS doctorate which has emerged in the USA, and in South Africa traditional doctorates have included self-managed distance modules, while in Scandinavia thesis by publication is common.

References

Advisory Board for the Research Councils (1993). *The nature of the PhD: A discussion document*. London: Advisory Board for the Research Councils.

Anderson, C. A. (2000). Current strengths and limitations of doctoral education in nursing: Are we prepared for the future? *Journal of Professional Nursing*, **16**(4), 191–200.

Blancett, S. S. (1989). Defining doctoral education. *Nurse Educator*, **14**, 3.

Bigbee, J. L. (1996). History and evolution of advanced nursing practice. In: A. B. Hamrick, J. A. Spross and C. M. Hanson (eds). *Advanced nursing practice: An integrative approach*. Philadelphia: Saunders, pp. 3–24.

Boore, J. R. P. (1996). Postgraduate education in nursing: A case study. *Journal of Advanced Nursing*, **23**, 620–629.

Boore, J. R. P. (1997). Doctoral level education in the health professions. *Teaching in Higher Education,* **1**(1), 29–48.

Booth, C. (2001). Broader PhD courses start at 10 universities. *Research Fortnight*, April 25, 2001. http://www.newphd.ac.uk (accessed on 05/06/04).

Bourner, T., Bowden, R. and Laing, S. (2001). Professional doctorates in England. *Studies in Higher Education,* **26**(1), 65–94.

Cotton, A. H. (1997). Power, knowledge and the discourse of specialisation in nursing. *Clinical Nurse Specialist,* **11**(1) 25–29.

Doncaster, K. and Thorne, L. (2000). Reflection and planning: Essential elements of professional doctorates. *Reflective Practice,* **1**(3), 391–399.

Downs, F. (1989). Differences between the professional doctorate and the academic/research doctorate. *Journal of Professional Nursing*, **5**, 261–265.

Flaherty, M. J. (1989). The doctor of nursing science degree: Evolutionary and societal perspectives. In: S. E. Hart (ed.). *Doctoral education in nursing: History, process, and outcomes.* New York: National League for Nursing, pp. 17–31.

Galvin, K. T. and Carr, E. (2002). The emergence of professional doctorates: Where are we now? Paper presented at the conference *Transforming Healthcare*, Trinity College, Dublin, November 2002.

Galvin, K. T. and Carr, E. (2003). The emergence of professional doctorates in nursing in the UK. Where are we now? *NTResearch*, **8**(4), 292–307.

Grypdonck, M. (2001). *Scholarship in nursing: How can PhD education contribute to its development?* Paper presented at the International Network for Doctoral Education in Nursing conference. Copenhagen, Denmark. Available at http://www.umich.edu/~inden/papers/ (accessed on 20.07.2003).

Higher Education Funding Council for England (2002). *Quality assurance assessment codes of practice*. Bristol: HEFCE.

Holloway, I. and Walker, J. (2000). *Getting a PhD in health and social care.* Oxford: Blackwell Science.

Hudacek, S. and Carpenter, D. R. (1998). Student perceptions of nurse doctorates: Similarities and differences. *Journal of Professional Nursing*, **14**(1), 14–21.

International Network for Doctoral Education in Nursing (2002). *Quality criteria and indicators of doctoral programs.* http://www.umich.edu/~inden/ (accessed on 05/06/04).

Ketefian, S., Neves, E. P. and Gutierrez, M. G. (2001). Nursing doctorate education in the Americas. *Online Journal of Issues in Nursing*, 5(2), 8.

Lancaster, L. E. (1984). Doctoral education in nursing, the Sisyphian concept, and Pandora's Box [Guest Editorial]. *Critical Care Nurse*, **4**(3), 6–17.

McKenna, H. and Cutcliffe, J. (2001). Nursing doctorate education in the United Kingdom and Ireland. *Online Journal of Issues in Nursing*, 5(2), 9.

Mason, C. and McKenna, H. P. (1995). How to survive a PhD. *Nurse Researcher* **2**(3), 73–79.

Murphy, J. (1981). Doctoral education *in*, *of*, and *for* nursing: An historical analysis. *Nursing Outlook*, **29**, 645–648.

Newman, M. (1975). The professional doctorate in nursing: Position paper. *Nursing Outlook*, **23**, 704–706.

Pearson, A., Borbasi, S., and Gott, M. (1997). Doctoral education in nursing for practitioner knowledge and for academic knowledge. *Journal of Nursing Scholarship*, **29**, 365–367.

Pickard, M. R. (1986). The non-traditional doctorate: An asset or liability in nursing education? *Nurse Educator*, **11**(6), 33.

Pierce, D. and Peyton, C. (1999). A historical cross-disciplinary perspective on the Professional Doctorate in Occupational Therapy. *American Journal of Occupational Therapy*, **53**, 64–71.

Queensland University of Technology (2003). *PhD Regulations Section 14: Presentation of PhD Theses by Published Work*. www.research.qut.edu.au/restdncen/postgraduate.jsp (accessed on 05/06/04).

Sakalys, J. A. Coates, C. J. and Chinn, P. L. (1995). Doctoral education in nursing: Evaluation of a non-traditional program option. *Journal of Professional Nursing*, **11**(5), 281–289.

Scott, P. A. and Conrad, C. F. (1992). A critique of intensive courses and an agenda for research. In: J. C. Smart (ed.). *Higher Education: Handbook of Theory and Research*, **8**, 411–459. New York, NY: Agathon Press.

Seitz, P. (1987). The pros and cons of doctoral education. *The Canadian Nurse*, **83**, 27.

Traynor, M. and Rafferty, A. M. (1998). *Nursing research and the higher education context*. A second working paper. London: Centre for Policy in Nursing Research, London School of Hygiene and Tropical Medicine.

UK Council for Graduate Education (2002). *Professional Doctorates*. Dudley: England.

Utrecht University (2003). Doctoral degree (PhD). Available at: http://www.uu.nl/phd (accessed on 05.06.2003).

Ziemer, M., Brown, J., Fitzpatrick, M. L., Manfriedi, C., O'Leary, J. and Valiga, T.M. (1992). Doctoral programs in nursing: Philosophy, curricula, and program requirements. *Journal of Professional Nursing*, **8**, 56–62.

Chapter 11

Models of international exchange for doctoral students and faculty

Hugh P. McKenna, Shaké Ketefian and Ann Whall

It is a truism, but the oft-repeated phrase 'the world is getting smaller' is an accurate reflection of reality. The Concorde could cross the Atlantic at twice the speed of sound, an e-mail message can be written in London and be read in Tokyo within seconds, and a person in northern China can see and speak to a colleague in Iceland using modern cell phone technology. There are hundreds of similar examples all showing that technology has contributed to the shrinking of our planet.

Nursing is a profession that has a worldwide presence and its members have consistently tried to bridge the knowledge and geographical boundaries that separate them. Florence Nightingale learned her nursing skills in Kaiserswerth in Germany and in Dublin in Ireland. She travelled with other nurses to Scutari in Turkey to nurse the sick and wounded of the Crimean War. On her return to London, she founded St Thomas' School of Nursing that acted as the distributing point for graduating nurses to take up prestigious posts in various parts of the world.

Ogilvie et al (2003) have argued that the development of international nursing requires a global focus and international collaboration. Today, nurses continue to link internationally with the objectives of exchanging ideas and working together for the benefits of patients, families and communities. A widely recognized advantage of successful internationalization is the improved access to knowledge and information. In nursing, global communication has increased through such means as print journals, electronic journals, e-learning materials, international conference proceedings, visiting scholar schemes, videoconferencing, internet discussion groups, and faculty and student exchanges. Such worldwide dissemination of nursing knowledge and information represents a novel opportunity to expand the reach and impact of professional nursing (Dougherty et al, 2004).

According to Francis (1993), internationalization is a process that prepares the nursing community for successful participation in an increasingly interdependent research world. This process should infuse all facets of the education system, fostering global sharing, understanding, and developing knowledge and skills for effective care in a diverse world.

More recently, the World Health Organization (1996) stated that nursing has the potential to make a positive contribution to global health. In the same year the Council of Europe called for joint projects that would benefit healthcare in European countries. More specifically, according to Hegyvary (2001) international collaboration provides alternative modes of thinking for nursing scholars, enables wide-range testing of theories in practice, facilitates scholarly maturity through self-assessment, and leads to the advancement of nursing science.

Dougherty et al (2004) maintain that international collaborations are important because they improve our knowledge and understanding of human needs across geographic boundaries, support a global perspective for nursing by fostering a worldwide inclusiveness; and expand the cultural and ethical values underpinning the goals in nursing.

Nonetheless, international collaboration, while enjoyable and fruitful, is hard work and a great deal of meticulous planning is required to achieve success. One of the first issues that needs to be addressed is to identify with the 'who', 'where' and 'why' of collaboration. If people are going to invest time and effort in collaboration, then selectivity and focus are key principles to consider. Initially they may spend time finding out where the required expertise exists and if these experts are interested in collaboration. As with all things, this is easier if funding is available.

Collaborations require careful nurturing. They soon cease if one partner perceives that they are contributing more than anyone else and getting little in return. There should be a strategic plan and the aims of the collaboration need to be agreed at the outset through a 'Memorandum of Understanding' (MoU) or a mutually agreed contract. Included in such documents should be agreement on intellectual property rights emanating from the collaboration and agreements on publication and conference presentation protocols. The MoU should also outline the commitment required of each organization and the people involved. It is recommended that prospective partners explore options before getting involved too quickly or too intensely. It is not unusual for a partner to think they are getting involved in a research collaboration when in fact the main focus of the project may be education. It is also important to realize that a high profile nursing school should balance carefully its national and international linkages. It would not be beneficial to a school's profile if it was well known for its expertise in Ghana but not in the local clinics or neighbouring health facilities in its home country.

Cultural imperialism, claims of methodological superiority, and language difficulties can impede collaboration. A country or school of nursing should not be judged by its weaknesses but by its strengths. Collaborators, especially from developed countries, must have cultural sensitivity where they think globally and value diversity. In many cases it is beneficial to learn a new language and develop an attitude of partnership and collaboration. It is common sense not to compete with existing programmes. Ways of identifying such programmes include enquiring through funding agencies and professional nursing organizations. It is often a good idea to build on international relationships that already exist or work with others in one's own organization that have existing strong international collaborations and relationships.

One area that is having significant impact internationally has to do with the initiatives being taken by individuals and institutions across the world. This is an area where institutional leaders are manifesting a great deal of creativity. Typically, this type of initiative is built on pre-existing individual relationships, where an institution approaches another to develop either a formal or informal partnership. The initiating individual will present the type of objective his/her institution would like to meet, and what their aspirations are in such a relationship. Thus begins a dialogue in which both parties begin clarifying what goals to pursue, what activities are feasible in the short term and in the long term, and begin developing strategies for achieving them.

Such alignments may occur between and among institutions that are 'equals' in their standing or on the developmental stage, or it may occur between an institution that is less developed and one that has more to offer. Invariably, however, as receptivity of the parties grows to these types of relationship, parties begin to see the strengths that reside in each other, and ways in which both can be enriched by collaborating through a variety of faculty and student exchange relationships. The ways in which each party might benefit from such arrangements are likely to be different, but the opportunities for mutual enrichment are invariably present.

In such instances one has to leave the door open to allow a variety of approaches to emerge, and not aim for each party to do the same thing in the exchange relationship. For example, one institution may wish to send a faculty member to the partner school to work with a colleague to hone research skills and collaborate on research, while the latter might send a doctoral student to the former school to work with a faculty specialist to help refine the dissertation ideas or to learn a particular design or the application of an instrument or a specific analytic technique. Similarly, in a given year an institution may not have a particular need and may not send someone to the partner school, while the other may do so. The extent of the activities need not be equal or parallel in every instance.

A major issue in such instances is funding. Experience shows that several approaches have been used. Some individuals are able to apply to a governmental or private funding agency to facilitate study overseas; others may be able to use a sabbatical period to accomplish the international visit, while others may already have research funding and are able to use such funds to meet expenses.

The number of funding organizations that support international nursing collaborations has increased in recent years. They are too numerous to name and there is always a strong possibility of inadvertently excluding some in an international text. In the rest of this chapter we will describe different models illustrating some ongoing collaborations.

Government-funded model

EU–USA exchange programmes

Each year the European Union (EU) in Brussels, Belgium, and the United States Department of Education in Washington, USA, fund collaborative projects. Several of these have been and continue to be focused on nursing. Normally, the projects have a three-year lifespan and on the EU side of the project there should be partners in at least three different countries whereas on the US side of the project there should be partners in at least three different states. At the core of all the projects is student and faculty exchange between the EU and the USA. For example, one of the authors of this chapter has been involved in two EU–USA projects. One focuses on nursing care for older people and the partners are: Kalmer University in Sweden, the University of Ulster in Northern Ireland, the University of Padua in Italy, the University of East Tennessee, Hampton College in Virginia and Otterbein University in Ohio. Each year for three years students and faculty from the US partners spend time (eight weeks) studying in Europe and vice versa. Such exchanges lead to joint publications from a common data set, and further research and education collaborations.

Brussels provides funding for the European partners and Washington funds the US partners. However, the funds are nominal and it is expected that the partner institutions contribute to the cost of the projects. This is mainly done through releasing and supporting faculty to participate. Because this is public money, both the EU and US funders require regular and often bureaucratic reports on progress. Nonetheless, these programmes have been so successful that recently similar programmes have been established between the EU and Canada and the EU and South Africa.

National Institute of Cancer consortia

The National Institute of Cancer (NCI) is a federally funded organization based within the National Institutes of Health at Bethesda in Maryland, USA. Through forming consortia with overseas governments, it opens its courses and wide range of expertise to nurses in other countries. In October 1999 it established an international consortium to promote the most effective preventative and therapeutic strategies for the management of cancer care through:

- Clinical trials training
- Predoctoral fellowships
- Clinical oncology nurse training
- Summer genetics seminars through the National Institute of Nursing Research
- NCI summer curriculum in cancer prevention

The Cancer Nurses Consortium Working Group was established as a subgroup of the main Board, and is a link between NCI, the UK and Ireland. Its purpose was to facilitate and assist in implementing educational opportunities for nurses identified under the consortium. It aimed to:

- promote an understanding of the consortium activities among nurses and encourage participation
- design and assist in implementing agreed-upon education and research programmes approved under a memorandum of understanding and to address local cancer strategies when necessary and appropriate
- identify and make recommendations for future development needs
- identify obstacles and recommend strategies to overcome them
- provide 'programme content' for general promotion of consortium activities, including the website and newsletter
- monitor activities in the nursing arena and report on progress to the consortium Board.

Under the aegis of the working group two cancer nursing PhD fellowships are available. A core element of these three-year full-time fellowships is that each fellow spends one year at the NCI in Bethesda. Each fellow would receive £25,000 per year plus travel and accommodation expenses. The working group also provides funding for nurses to go to the NCI to attend short courses in clinical trials, ethics and cancer prevention. These short courses are typically 12 weeks in length, and a number of oncology nurses have achieved successful completion.

Membership model

European Academy of Nursing Science

The European Academy of Nursing Science (EANS) was established in 1999 to enhance scholarship and nursing science in Europe. It is an independently organized body composed of individual members who have made significant contributions to the advancement of nursing science in Europe through scholarship and research. The purpose of the Academy is to sustain a forum of European nurse scientists to develop and promote knowledge in nursing science and to recognize research and scholarly achievement in the pursuit of excellence. The principal activities of the Academy concern the advancement of nursing science through annual meetings of the fellows and honorary fellows of the Academy, and scientific and educational activities through the provision of advice on all matters concerning the development of nursing science in Europe.

A core aspect of the EANS business is the European Network of Doctoral Nursing Programmes. This offers the opportunity to add a European dimension to a doctoral research project. The aims of the programme are:

- to provide a common European perspective for doctoral nursing research
- to create a multinational learning environment for doctoral students in nursing
- to enhance the opportunities for doctoral students to study
- to develop a network in a European perspective.

This is a three-year programme. The first year incorporates a 10-day intensive course, whereas years 2 and 3 include a one-week course. Readers can gain an overview of the programme by studying an outline of the 2002 course taught in Edinburgh (www.omv.lu.se/bill001/eans).

International Network of Doctoral Education in Nursing (http://www.umich.edu/~inden)

The International Network for Doctoral Education in Nursing (INDEN) aims to advance and promote high quality doctoral education in nursing through national and international collaboration. Its goal is to become a major facilitator worldwide for achieving exchange of faculty and students across countries and programmes. There are many avenues through which this goal can be pursued and the initial step has been to organize doctoral student seminars in different parts of the world through collaboration with international institutions.

For the first seminar of this type, INDEN collaborated with the universities of Melbourne, Australia, and Michigan, USA, to offer a one-week seminar on the campus of the University of Melbourne, with both institutions providing faculty experts. The seminar was announced to all INDEN members, along with guidelines for submission of applications. A selection committee reviewed the applicants and 12 students representing seven countries were admitted to the programme. The initial focus of the seminar was on children and adolescents. It was soon realized that this was a very narrow theme, and the interests of applicant students were broader than the desire to learn about a particular clinical area. Students were interested in meeting colleagues from different countries, learning about how doctoral education was organized and taught, how to move through different phases of doctoral study, learn about how faculty go about developing a programme of research throughout their careers, and to discuss methodological options for their dissertation.

The second international student seminar was also a collaborative effort – between INDEN and an existing consortium of four international universities (see the Four Country Project later in this chapter). This seminar was hosted by the Department of Nursing at Lund University, Sweden, in 2003. INDEN was invited to send four students to join the faculty/student seminar. Each institution had sent several faculty and student members. Both doctoral students and faculty presented their research work in the area of chronic illness, followed by indepth discussion on theoretical, methodological and ethical issues related to the presentation. The students found these to be very enriching and enlightening. The students were pursuing diverse areas of research with the larger theme of chronic illness, and proposing different methodological approaches (examples of chronic conditions that were considered are depression, cognitive dysfunctions among the elderly, and cardiac problems).

The students prepared a collective paper for the INDEN electronic *Newsletter*, in which they summarized the multiple ways in which the experience was enriching for them. These included broadening their perspectives on chronic illness and the issues to be considered in research; providing an opportunity to network and exchange ideas with other doctoral students; exploring the potential for international collaborative research programmes which would assist in developing culturally sensitive nursing practice; and the enhancement of critical thinking and academic discourse. This enabled the students to receive input from individuals from different parts of the world, providing them with new ways of looking at issues. They felt they experienced support and respect for their work and an increased awareness about various considerations that researchers must pay attention to when selecting a particular methodological approach.

INDEN expects to build on this beginning and to continue collaborating with institutions in these efforts. Another focus that is emerging, and related to this initiative for doctoral students, is the facilitation of faculty exchange opportunities. Preliminary and foundational work is necessary before this initiative can get under way. A database needs to be created on what various institutions are offering by way of faculty expertise and collaborative research. The database needs to include institutional profile, faculty profiles and student profiles. A system needs to be put in place to facilitate matching existing opportunities with individual needs, and assisting with a search for resources to bring about the exchange (this effort is now under way by INDEN). Some of this has begun to happen. Faculty from some countries are seeking to make direct contacts with institutions and published scholars to spend their sabbatical periods collaborating on research. These faculty members are typically in mid-career, seeking to recharge themselves with new ideas and interactions with established scholars or begin new areas of research. They tend to be supported by their own institutions. A number of research-intensive universities in the USA are host to this type of faculty exchange programmes. Informal evaluations in several settings reveal that both parties find this enriching, leading to collaborative research in the years to come.

Another example of student exchange that has emerged has been stimulated by the needs in some countries and is referred to as the 'sandwich' programme. Some countries that are newly developing doctoral education find that students are enriched by spending a year overseas in the middle of their study to engage in a variety of supervised activities on a research-intensive campus. This is felt to be less costly than sending students overseas for their entire study period.

Some students spend the year developing their dissertation proposals; some engage in research with faculty and some do combinations of the two activities. Alternatively, if a student has not been able to engage in this type of international study during their doctorate, their employer sends them overseas for one year of postdoctorate study focusing exclusively on research, prior to beginning their formal employment as faculty members.

Independent models

Harkness Fellowship in healthcare policy

Each year the Commonwealth Fund, New York, supports ten Harkness fellows to study for one year in the USA. The competition is open to the UK, Australia and New Zealand. In the main, these are postdoctoral fellowships and focus on any aspect of healthcare policy. They provide a unique opportunity for promising health policy researchers and practitioners (e.g. nurses, physicians, health services managers) who are early in their career to spend four to 12 months in the USA conducting a policy-oriented research project and working with leading US health policy experts.

Fellows must demonstrate a strong interest in health policy issues and propose a well-designed research study that falls within the scope of the Fund's national programme areas. These are: improving healthcare services; improving the health of minorities; advancing the wellbeing of elderly people; and developing the capacities of children and young people.

Studies that include comparisons between the USA and the applicant's home country are encouraged. The Fund provides extensive support to successful fellows to help them develop and shape their research proposals to fit the US context. Through its extensive network of contacts, the Fund helps identify and place each fellow with a mentor who is an expert in the area to be studied. Fellows are also required to identify a home country mentor, who will liaise with the US mentor and supervise any cross-national comparisons that are to be conducted as part of the study.

Each fellowship provides up to US$75,000 in support, which includes round trip airfare to the USA, a monthly stipend, support towards any portion of the study conducted in the home country, project-related travel and other research expenses, tuition for related academic courses, and health insurance. In addition, a family supplement is available to fellows accompanied by a spouse and/or children.

Florence Nightingale Foundation Travel Scholarship

The Florence Nightingale Travel Scholarship supports a number of nurses to travel to other countries. These scholarships are prestigious and have resulted in the exchange of ideas and practices between nurses across the world. They are available to all British and Commonwealth nurses. They are awarded for projects connected with the applicant's field of work and which will benefit their patients/clients and the profession more widely. Candidates should have at least two years' professional experience subsequent to registration. Applications from those nurses who are at the developmental stage of their career are particularly welcome. In particular, doctoral students can use the Scholarship to visit a subject or methodology expert in another country.

Fulbright Scholars Program

The US senator J. William Fulbright was so devastated by the destruction he saw during the Second World War, that he came to believe that wars might be averted by closer communication to produce better and clearer 'mutual understandings' between the countries of the world. As a result Senator Fulbright initiated the Fulbright Program, sponsored by the US Department of State and the Bureau of Educational and Cultural Affairs; similar entities provide Fulbright support in countries around the world. The Fulbright stands as a vital link between academic, professional and personal (relationships) between 144 countries throughout the world. The Fulbright programme has so far supported more than 200,000 persons in its more than half century of existence. It has come to be recognized as a pre-eminent academic vehicle for international understanding and joint international initiatives.

Upon initial review, Fulbright programmes appear very complex, in that they are multiple and variable. With greater understanding, however, it becomes clear that this complexity has led to a flexibility that makes possible the overall success of the programme. Fulbright programmes have an underlying stability of structure, although various aspects of the programmes are modified yearly to meet the changing characteristics of both the applicants as well as the Fulbright goals.

The statement that the Fulbright programme 'supports outstanding graduate students, researchers, and established leaders of professional, academic, and artistic excellence', identifies the bifurcation of the award structure into awards to promising students as well as awards to established academics. The awards are further divided in that support from both a home and host academic institution is required. This requirement bespeaks the necessity of designing a plan of work for the Fulbright effort that meets the goals at both institutions. Although a Fulbright catalogue of possible host institutions is available that advertises desired areas of work, the absence of an institution from this list should not dissuade applicants. Host institutions not listed in this catalogue are often sought out by applicants using advice of colleagues as to the excellence of the work being done in the area of the applicant's interest. The excellence of the work plus the willingness of a principal at a host institution to assist in both designing the Fulbright plan as well as providing the necessary letters of support and other documentation for the Fulbright application is of the greatest importance.

An additional feature of Fulbright programmes is a general willingness on the part of various Fulbright commissions throughout the world to consider important but unrecognized and thus non-described types of activity someone might wish to pursue via Fulbright support. Host institutions and the Fulbright review committee are also willing to accept plans of varying lengths of time, if both the host and home schools are agreeable. Such characteristics of Fulbright support are wonderful as well as somewhat confusing to a new applicant. As with any vital organization, however, this 'confusion quotient' is in a sense the price one must pay if one wishes to participate.

For these reasons, anyone wishing to undertake a project supported by Fulbright must not only consult current descriptions of available programmes, but it is also wise to telephone or otherwise personally interact with the person identified within Fulbright materials as representing a particular programme. This personal contact should be used not only to clarify specific questions, but also to check current Fulbright thinking regarding continuing support for a given mechanism. Information regarding current levels of financial support for specific programmes is usually best accessed in this way. Support varies from country to country but generally includes travel funds and some basic maintenance allowance.

It is useful to access Fulbright information for one's home country as well as that for the country in which Fulbright activities might be carried out. The web address www.cies.org (Council for the International Exchange of Scholars) provides general information on current programmes available, likewise the address www.Fulbright.org contains additional information. The major US Fulbright programmes available as of November, 2003 that can be downloaded directly from the CIES website, are as follows:

- Traditional Fulbright Scholar Program: the traditional Fulbright Scholar Program sends 800 US faculty and professionals abroad to 140 countries each year for two months to an academic year. Grantees lecture and conduct research in a wide variety of academic and professional fields.
- Fulbright Distinguished Chairs Program: the Fulbright Distinguished Chairs Program awards are among the most prestigious appointments in the Fulbright Scholar Program. Most awards are in Western Europe, although a few are available in Canada and Russia.
- Fulbright Senior Specialists Program: the Fulbright Senior Specialists Program provides short-term Fulbright grants of two to six weeks. Activities offer US faculty and professionals opportunities to collaborate on curriculum and faculty development, institutional planning and a variety of other activities.
- Fulbright New Century Scholars Program: 30 top academics and professionals collaborate for a year on a topic of global significance. For 2002–2003, the research theme was 'Addressing sectarian, ethnic and cultural conflict within and across national borders'.

- Fulbright Alumni Initiatives Awards Program: this programme offers small institutional grants to Fulbright alumni to continue or develop projects that will link their home and host institutions.

In addition, those who have been US Fulbright awardees (or 'Fulbrighters') are invited to join the Fulbright Association, a membership organization of Fulbright alumni and supporters committed to fostering international awareness and understanding through advocating increased worldwide support for Fulbright exchanges, enriching the Fulbright experience and facilitating lifelong interaction among alumni and current participants.

Self-funded model

Four Country Project

In 2000 the deans of nursing from the University of North Carolina at Chapel Hill, North Carolina, USA, and the University of Ulster in Northern Ireland, UK, agreed to set up faculty and doctoral student collaboration. Each agreed to involve another partner with which they were already collaborating and this resulted in the University of Lund in Sweden and the University of Toronto in Canada joining a collaboration called the Four Country Project.

Every year, one of the partners hosts a five-day research workshop on a theme of relevance to a cadre of faculty and doctoral students in all four institutions. The other three partners send students and faculty to participate in the workshop. For example, in the year 2001, the University of North Carolina at Chapel Hill hosted a workshop on maternal and child health. The universities of Ulster, Lund and Toronto sent doctoral students (three to four each) and faculty (two to three each). The workshop involves presentations from students on their doctoral studies and on methodological issues, talks by faculty participants and guest speakers who are experts on the theme. An important aspect of the workshop is the social events where students and faculty get to know each other and cement further research alliances.

The funding model of the Four Country Project is simple. The host institution arranges the event and guest speakers and supplies the accommodation and social calendar for the incoming students and faculty. The visiting institutions meet the travel and food expenses. This means that every four years an institution has to organize the event and arrange accommodation. In 2002 the event was held at the University of Ulster and the theme was research on care of older people. In 2003, the University of Lund hosted the event and the theme was research on living with chronic illness. The University of Toronto will host the 2004 event.

University of Michigan Project

It is not a blinding insight to posit that collaboration and exchanges occur and build on existing relationships. Individuals would like to collaborate with those whom they know, have developed a professional or personal relationship with, and have formed the basis for trust. For example, if one were to enquire about how various institutional partnerships and relationships came to be, one would find that someone from institution A went to graduate school with someone in institution B; or that someone in institution A was the mentor for someone in institution B and supervised the person's dissertation. These are naturally excellent foundations on which to begin building. In a similar vein, anecdotal evidence shows that upon completion of a collaborative venture, there is much follow-on activity and various types of institutional relationships develop between the partners.

In the absence of these, opportunities can be created to lay the foundation for scholars to meet and begin the process of sharing and getting to know one another's work. Towards this end, the University of Michigan initiated a programme in 2003. The steps taken were as follows:

1 An invitation was sent to the faculty of the University of Michigan to indicate their interest in collaboratively working with international colleagues for an intensive week over the summer period. This solicitation specified that there needed to be a faculty research team in place that was developing programmatic research, with the team having at least one senior investigator along with other faculty and doctoral students or postdoctoral fellows on the team. The team was asked to send the research theme of interest to it.
2 The solicitation yielded six volunteer research teams that met the specifications.
3 A letter of invitation, in which the six research themes were listed, was sent to a number of international institutions. The letter invited these schools to nominate one faculty member (senior or junior) whose research was in one of the six identified areas. The letter identified the goal of the week-long workshop as aiming to initiate international research collaboration among the respective faculties. In sending a faculty member, the institution made a commitment to facilitate the person's collaborative research upon her or his return home, in terms of time provided for the collaboration or in facilitating the search for funding sources from the home country and the region.
4 A selection process was undertaken, with the senior faculty member from each of the six teams participating. The nominations and the supporting materials were so superb and so carefully presented that the team focused mainly on identifying those that presented the best fit with the research being conducted at Michigan.

5 This process yielded 11 scholars who visited the University of Michigan for seven days. Their institutions paid for travel, and the University of Michigan paid for room and board.

Most of the week-long workshop was spent in intensive work among the small groups with one of the six research teams. Each team had one to four individuals assigned. The teams assumed responsibility for how the time would be spent, but in all cases, there was sharing of one another's research programmes and work to date, and discussion on the theoretical foundations and specific methodologic approaches used. There were some site visits to agencies to see specific patient populations, appointments with other experts in the area or within the institution, or demonstration of how specific interventions were applied.

At the end of each day all visiting scholars convened together for a final session and a special presentation/discussion was planned. These included an overview of proposal preparation, how to conceptualize a research problem and develop a theoretical rationale, and an overview of international funding sources. Evenings were spent as social time with dinners hosted by various faculty and administrators of the host institution.

Some teams actually used the week to prepare a collaborative research proposal, while others used the time to re-think their direction and committed themselves to start proposal preparation upon return home. Many of the teams are in continuing contact as to their next steps.

Visiting faculty were overwhelmingly positive, pointing to the workshop as a time to get away from daily commitments and to think only about nursing research; some stated that their horizons were broadened and that they developed new insights and new ways of seeing the problem of interest; many expressed the view that without this opportunity they would not have been able to begin the process of international collaboration.

The group as a whole noted with great satisfaction that it was a unique opportunity for them to get to know and share views with the other participants from the seven different countries, and there was some discussion among them regarding future individual collaborations. They expressed appreciation to the faculty of the host school for their dedication to the entire process.

The faculty of the University of Michigan similarly were pleased and expressed the hope that there will be concrete outcomes as follow-up. They did point to the fact that it was hard work, yet highly worthwhile. A number of teams had doctoral students participating in the discussions. Some of these students had previously not had the opportunity to work with international scholars and pointed to the personal and professional enrichment this brought to their scholarly work.

At the time of writing one proposal had been submitted by a team; in the case of another team, discussions were under way for a visiting scholar to send a doctoral student to work and study with the team she herself worked with to facilitate the student's dissertation proposal development. This is a most promising beginning a few months after the end of the workshop. Time will tell what other follow-on collaborative projects will evolve. We do know from the evaluations that a good foundation has been provided on which to build. Should circumstances allow, a repeat will be considered in several years, inviting several of the scholars from the first workshop and adding new individuals to the group.

Summary and conclusion

As stated at the outset of this chapter, it is incumbent upon the nursing profession to share expertise and experiences internationally. Morally, best practice should be available to all the citizens of this planet and collaborations assist in disseminating best practices. With technology making the world a smaller place, collaboration is easier than it has been hitherto. There are many opportunities for nurses to bridge the knowledge and geographical gaps that continue to exist. This chapter has outlined a small number of these collaborations reflecting different models including government-funded models (EU–US Project; National Cancer Institute consortia), membership models (EANS; INDEN), independent models (Harkness, Fulbright, Nightingale Fellowship) and self-funding models (Four Country Project, University of Michigan Project). Each of these models supports the exchange of students and faculty and enhances the knowledge base of the discipline. The above models were presented as examples only, and were not meant to be an exhaustive list of all the opportunities that are available. In addition to the existing programmes for faculty and student exchange opportunities that the interested person can investigate, there is room for creativity, whereby individuals and institutions can create models and programmes best suited for the goals at hand.

References

Dougherty, M. C., Lin, S. Y., McKenna, H. P. and Seers, K. (2004). International content of high-ranking nursing journals in the year 2000. *Journal of Nursing Scholarship*, **36**(2), 173–179.

European Academy of Nursing Science (EANS) (2004). www.omv.lu.se/bill001/eans (accessed on 02.05.04).

Francis, A. (1993). *Facing the future: The internationalization of post-secondary institutions in British Columbia. Task Force Report.* Vancouver: Columbia Centre for International Education.

Fulbright Fellowships. www.cies.org (accessed on 02/05/04). www.Fulbright.org (accessed on 02.05/04).

Hegyvary, S. T. (2001). The importance of context. *Journal of Nursing Scholarship,* **33**(1), 4.

International Network of Doctoral Education in Nursing (2004). University of Michigan, Ann Arbor, USA. http://www.umich.edu/~inden (accessed on 02/05/04).

Ogilvie, L., Allen, M., Laryea, J. and Opare, M. (2003). Building capacity through a collaborative international nursing project. *Journal of Nursing Scholarship,* **35**(2), 113–118.

World Health Organization (1996). *Nursing Practice.* WHO Technical Report, series 860. Geneva, Switzerland: WHO.

Chapter 12

Postdoctoral study: bridging the gap to independent scientist

Carol Loveland-Cherry and Kobkul Phancharoenworakul

In the USA, postdoctoral preparation has developed over the past approximately 100 years in response to the need for additional research training (American Association of Universities [AAU], 1998). The Johns Hopkins University initiated postdoctoral preparation shortly after its founding in 1876 and the Rockefeller Foundation established formal postdoctoral fellowships for recent PhD graduates in the physical sciences at the beginning of the twentieth century. Postdoctoral preparation grew modestly in the first half of the past century, but increased rapidly in the 1970s.

The US federal government has supported predoctoral and postdoctoral preparation for nurses since 1955 (Hinshaw and Lucas, 1993). Postdoctoral preparation in nursing has a history that parallels that of doctoral education, but beginning at a later time. Until there was a critical body of nurses prepared at the doctoral level, there was not great demand for postdoctoral training opportunities. In nursing, the first doctoral programmes were initiated at Teachers College, Columbia University, in 1933 and at New York University in 1934 (Fisher and Habermann, 2000). By 2003, there were approximately 273 doctoral programmes in nursing across the world (INDEN, 2003). The largest numbers of programmes are located in the Americas, followed by the European Region, and then the Asian/Pacific Region (see Table 12.1).

It is difficult to ascertain the number of nurses in postdoctoral study from a national or international perspective. The number of postdoctoral fellows reported in the annual American Association of Colleges of Nursing survey was 66 for 2002, a decrease from 70 in 2001 (Berlin, Stennett and Bednash, 2002–2003). Initially, mentors for postdoctoral opportunities for nurses primarily were in other related disciplines, such as psychology, sociology, physiology, public health and education. As a cadre of active nurse researchers was established, postdoctoral training within the nursing discipline became viable.

Doctoral study is an intense experience that provides students basic preparation in knowledge development through a variety of research and theory development approaches. Additionally, students need to develop indepth knowledge within a specific content area. Ideally, doctoral study would prepare scholars who are ready to launch independent research programmes (Wood, 2002).

Table 12.1 International nursing doctoral programmes

Location	*Number*	*Percentage*
Argentina	2	0.7
Australia	15	5.5
Belgium	4	1.5
Brazil	9	3.3
Canada	11	4.0
Chile	1	0.36
Colombia	1	0.36
Czech Republic	4	1.5
Egypt	7	2.6
Finland	6	2.2
Germany	3	1.1
Greece	1	0.36
Hong Kong	3	1.1
Ireland	3	1.1
Japan	9	3.3
Korea	12	4.4
Mexico	1	0.36
Namibia	1	0.36
The Netherlands	4	1.5
New Zealand	2	0.7
Norway	3	1.1
Philippines	3	1.1
Poland	1	0.36
South Africa	10	3.7
Sweden	8	2.9
Taiwan	3	1.1
Thailand	6	2.2
Turkey	6	2.2
United Kingdom	52	19.0
United States of America	81	29.6
Venezuela	1	0.36
Total	273	

Note
Adapted from data from the International Network for Doctoral Education in Nursing, http://www.umich.edu/~inden/programs/, accessed 25.12.2003).

However, the timelines, coursework and dissertation deadlines make it difficult for doctoral students to develop these skills in great depth (Paul, 2000) in the 'taught' model of doctoral education (McKenna, 2000) common in the USA and other parts of the world. The British/European model of doctoral education is structured as a research mentorship with minimal coursework. Within the latter model, the focus is on research with less emphasis on building a knowledge base for the discipline (McKenna, 2000). Within either model, the doctoral programme merely provides the foundation for developing as an independent researcher. The key to success relies on the postdoctoral fellowship. Although many individuals can succeed without this additional preparation, most people would benefit from the additional preparation (Wood, 2002). For some disciplines, such as biochemistry and physics, the postdoctoral fellowship 'has become the *de facto* terminal academic credential' (AAU, 2003, p. 1).

Postdoctoral training helps consolidate the academic skills and scholarly habits needed to prepare for a postdoctoral fellow's long-term career plans. It is a period in which researchers develop a 'specialized, focused area of both substantive content and methodological strategies' (Hinshaw and Lucas, 1993, p. 309). A postdoctoral training period helps the scholar to launch his or her long-term research focus before taking up the demands of academic teaching, service and tenure (Paul, 2000) and establish the basis of the research programme before taking up the demands of academic teaching and service, in addition to research. It should be designed to help a person develop skills and research expertise in a specific area (Lowe et al, 1991 as cited in Paul, 2000). In addition, tangible outcomes can include publications and preparation of a proposal that can be submitted for funding.

Career trajectories of doctorally prepared nurses

Similar to other disciplines, nurses who have completed their doctorate pursue a number of career options. Most doctorally prepared nurses take positions in research-intensive and teaching-intensive academic institutions. Although a large number of academic positions are tenure-track ones, a growing number of doctorally prepared nurses are choosing to move into non-tenure positions such as primary research scientist or lecturer positions. Generally, they are in high demand, unlike a number of other disciplines and they often have multiple offers of positions. The current faculty shortage in the USA has exacerbated this situation and new PhD graduates as well as experienced doctorally prepared faculty are in even higher demand than previously. In addition to faculty positions these individuals often hold responsible positions in the government, consulting firms, healthcare service organizations, and/or a professional association (in both the government and private sector). However, the majority of these individuals will work as faculty members at universities throughout the country and worldwide. Academic career pathways can vary across the world, but typically begin as a senior lecturer or assistant professor, advancing to associate professor and full professor. These positions are awarded depending on the applicant's research, teaching, and publications. As faculty members, they teach in the undergraduate, Master's and doctoral programmes, as well as develop their own research programmes.

In Thailand, some doctorally prepared nurses work at the Ministry of Public Health in the office of planning, policy and in the nursing department. They are involved in establishing health policies and developing the strategies needed to improve the quality of nursing care. The career pathways relate to the position classification beginning with C7 and going through C10. These positions will be awarded depending on the clinical research.

In the USA, doctorally prepared nurses are recruited into government positions at all levels and across agencies. At the state level, nurses are often employed in departments of public health to plan, implement, and evaluate intervention programmes, and to work on health policy. At the national level, the National Institutes of Health employ a number of nurses in both extramural and intramural programmes across its various institutes. Their positions range from managing clinical studies to directing and staffing the National Institute of Nursing Research. Other federal agencies, such as the Centers for Disease Control, employ doctorally prepared nurses in research and policy positions.

In the USA, clinical research positions for doctorally prepared nurses were developed in the 1980s and became fairly common. However, as hospitals, especially academic health centres where clinical nurse researchers were more likely to be employed, experienced financial difficulties, many of these positions were eliminated. Still other doctorally prepared nurses hold a variety of positions in healthcare institutions, including research and administrative positions. A growing number of nurse scientists are electing to combine research and practice in clinical faculty positions. Individuals in these positions, usually non-tenure track, are expected to generate support for their positions through clinical practice and research grants. Further, they may have some teaching and research mentoring responsibilities. In contrast, clinical research positions are not offered in Thai hospitals. However, the job description of the clinical nursing specialist in each hospital provides a cue that they have to conduct clinical research.

Although doctorally prepared nurses are in high demand and have considerable choices in selecting job options, those who assume faculty positions in research-intensive academic institutions often find that they are relatively disadvantaged in establishing a programme of research and meeting tenure criteria compared to colleagues who have had a postdoctoral experience. Successfully attaining tenure at research-intensive institutions requires that within five to seven years faculty need to have established a programme of research that is nationally and internationally recognized and preferably is externally funded. Research productivity must be accompanied by dissemination of scholarship results through publications and presentations. All this is to be done in addition to teaching and service activities. McGivern (2003, p. 60) cites Kohler (1990) as describing faculty 'not as professional researchers but as teachers who fit research into the small spaces of their career'.

Doctorally prepared nurses employed in service settings find that they need a repertoire of skills to assist with research needs of the institution with varied foci and may have limited time to focus on their own research. Postdoctoral preparation is one option available to nurse researchers to establish a research programme and solidify their research skills.

Structure and characteristics of postdoctoral study

As part of its report on postdoctoral education, the AAU (2003, p. 3) recommended the following definition of a postdoctoral experience:

- The appointee was recently awarded a PhD or equivalent doctorate (e.g. ScD, MD) in an appropriate field
- The appointment is temporary
- The appointment involves substantially full-time research or scholarship
- The appointment is viewed as preparatory for a full-time academic and/or research career
- The appointment is not part of a clinical training programme
- The appointee works under the supervision of a senior scholar or a department in a university or similar research institution (e.g. national laboratory, NIH) and
- The appointee has the freedom, and is expected, to publish the results of his or her research or scholarship during the period of the appointment.

There is no single structure for postdoctoral programmes. The goals of enhancing/augmenting research skills learned in a doctoral programme can be accomplished in a variety of ways. The AAU report (2003) highlighted the extreme flexibility and lack of policies for postdoctoral programmes. Postdoctoral appointments often have no limits, lack consistent campus-wide compensation policies, have limited formal job placement procedures, lack quality control, and depend on word of mouth recruitment.

In nursing, the structure of the postdoctoral experience also varies, depending on the source of funding and other factors. NIH institutional postdoctoral grants (T32), individual postdoctoral funding mechanisms (F32), and Career Development Awards (K01) provide more structure through the guidelines for these mechanisms. Applications for these awards require the formulation of clear goals and outcomes for the postdoctoral fellowship. The applicant is also required to identify specific activities and resources needed to support accomplishment of goals.

Generally, additional coursework is not a major focus and is, therefore, limited. The emphasis is on working with a mentor(s), presenting papers at scholarly meetings and publishing manuscripts based on the dissertation research or other recent work, attending interdisciplinary seminars on campus and scholarly conferences, conducting pilot research, developing a grant proposal for the next step in the programme of research, and meeting with other researchers (Albrecht and Greiner, 1992).

In order to accomplish the goals of the postdoctoral experience, there are specific resources that are needed. A research active mentor is critical to the success of postdoctoral work (Byrne and Keefe, 2003). Mentoring may require an additional co-mentor and access to consultants. As research becomes more interdisciplinary, the inclusion of co-mentors and consultants from other disciplines is common. Regular and focused interaction with the mentor(s) needs to be structured. Some additional coursework may be necessary to gain additional specific expertise needed for the identified area of research. Space, computer access and time are essential pragmatic resources. Finally, a productive research environment, preferably at an institution other than the one where the doctorate was earned, is needed to provide the context and resources to foster growth in research (Hinshaw and Lucas, 1993). In fact, Donaldson (2002) contends, 'The most important aspect of high-quality research training, whether pre- or postdoctoral, is the student's participation in an interactive, competitive, multidisciplinary research enterprise' (p. 1).

In nursing, the length of the postdoctoral fellowships generally is one to two years, with the preference being two years. Longer experiences are available depending upon the source of funding. For example, NIH K awards range from three to five years in length compared to one to two years for other mechanisms. The median duration of a postdoctoral fellowship is 2.5 years, but varies across disciplines from one year in engineering to 3.5–5 years in the life sciences and some physical sciences (Singer, 2000). In other disciplines, there are concerns about fellows remaining in postdoctoral positions for too long a period and having multiple postdoctoral appointments. In these situations, it may be the case that positions are not available in the fellow's field, and the postdoctorate serves as the 'employment'. These are not currently issues in nursing.

Application requirements vary across fellowships, but generally include a training plan, a research plan, description of the mentor, and a description of the research environment and resources. Supports for research, stipend, and benefits are generally available, but vary and are specific to the sources.

Current postdoctoral nursing programmes and opportunities

In the USA, a growing number of options are available and used by nurses to obtain postdoctoral preparation. A number of these opportunities are through specific funding mechanisms sponsored by governmental agencies, foundations, and professional organizations or private industry, such as pharmaceutical companies; individual researchers support others through their funded research projects. Consequently, there is no single published list of postdoctoral programmes. A recent online search for postdoctoral fellowships resulted in 94,200 hits and when limited to health, 51,600. Postdoctoral fellowships are concentrated in a small number of colleges and universities. Overall, approximately two-thirds of postdoctoral appointments are located in 50 of the nearly 350 doctorate-granting institutions (AAU, 2003). Among nursing schools, 25 of the 81 research doctoral programmes report offering postdoctoral study (Berlin et al, 2002–2003). Postdoctoral fellows also are located in other than academic institutions. While 80% are located in universities, 13% are in government and 7% in industrial settings (Singer, 2000).

The funding opportunities include both government and foundation sources, specific professional organizations and educational institutions, from around the world. Sorting through all of the potential sources is a challenging task. Trying to further specify the search to nursing was not fruitful. Clearly, not all of these sources may be open to nurse applicants, but as nurse scientists have gained stronger research preparation it is timely for them to apply to sources that are consistent with their research foci.

In the USA, the National Institutes of Health offer several funding mechanisms to support postdoctoral study. The options through the National Institute of Nursing Research include the Ruth L. Kirschstein Individual NRSA Postdoctoral Fellowships (F32), Senior NRSA Fellowship (F33), and Career Development Award (K award). The National Research Service Award Institutional Research Training Grant (T32) mechanism supports postdoctoral fellows, as well as predoctoral preparation. A listing of funding options and currently funded institutional predoctoral and postdoctoral programmes is available on the National Institute of Nursing Research's website, (http://www.nih.gov/ninr). The 27 institutional pre- and postdoctoral training grants listed include preparation across a variety of foci, including special populations such as women, children, families, elderly and across the spectrum of health promotion/risk reduction, and acute, and chronic illness. Most offer postdoctoral fellowships. Similar mechanisms are available through other NIH institutes and nurses have been successful in obtaining funding from a number of these institutes (e.g. National Institute on Aging, National Cancer Institute). The requirement of US citizenship/non-citizen nationals, or permanent residence limits these opportunities for international scholars. Other federal government fellowships are available from the Veterans Administration Postdoctoral Nurse Fellowship programme.

The Pfizer Postdoctoral Fellowship in Nursing Research: Innovations in Health Outcomes is an example of a non-governmental funding source. The programme is part of the Pfizer Medical and Academic Partnerships. The programme offers two postdoctoral fellowships each year. Applications include a training plan, a research plan, and identification of a mentor. This option allows an individual to be in a faculty position while holding the fellowship. Funding is for two years at US$130,000 per year. Fellows have flexibility in how the funds are used.

Advantages and challenges of postdoctoral study

There are several advantages and challenges to pursuing a postdoctoral fellowship. The advantages of a postdoctoral programme are not only for the individual but also for their employers and organizations, the nursing discipline, and finally the recipients of improved care. Postdoctoral fellowships are opportunities to develop both personally and professionally. The difficult work involved in pursuing a postdoctoral fellowship will almost certainly lead to the enhancement of the fellow's professional maturity, and often to personal growth as well. During postdoctoral training, a fellow has the unique opportunity to focus on one project. Their attention is not fragmented by the many other academic requirements such as teaching, administration, service and clinical practice. They are allowed to concentrate on their research, the writing of grants, publications, and presentations. This narrow focus is a valuable experience that is not always available to a doctoral student or new faculty members (Paul, 2002).

Lev et al (1990) have described postdoctoral fellowships as a way 'to offer the nurse investigator a number of experiences that may facilitate development as an independent investigator' (p. 116). Some nurses may choose a postdoctoral experience as a way of gaining additional research skills needed to change the direction of their research careers. Some postdoctoral programmes are specifically designed to prepare the fellow in areas perceived to be in need of researchers who can address specific research questions (Lev et al, 1990). The benefit to academic institutions is more well-prepared potential research faculty. Further, upon appointment to a faculty position, these individuals are less likely to need close supervision or mentoring, as they already have made a good start towards their programme of research.

Postdoctoral study should prepare scholars for employment as beginning independent researchers (Ketefian, 1991). These individuals can develop further as researchers in large research institutions, or can provide a solid base for research development in smaller colleges of nursing, hospitals or community health agencies (Albrecht and Greiner, 1992, p. 373). The emphasis on evidence-based practice and the nursing discipline's espoused value of the same, dictates that research is carried out to support this goal. Nurse scientists with postdoctoral training will be better prepared and positioned to contribute to the development of the knowledge base needed to support evidence-based practice in nursing. Contributions of postdoctoral fellows to the research and academic enterprises in the USA are significant; they conduct a significant portion of research in the country and provide additional research instruction to graduate students (AAU, 2003).

Challenges of postdoctoral study

There are a number of challenges to continuing in a postdoctoral programme including low pay, relocation, decreased status, career interruption and the absence of peers. These may produce stress, according to Chenitz and Swanson (1981). Financially, the postdoctoral programme can be a major setback for individuals. The funding award is often considerably less than the salary of a junior faculty member. Postdoctoral fellows frequently need to change location or institution, which takes them away from family and friends. They may encounter loneliness and social isolation. Leaving a faculty or other position requires managing the stress associated with a new environment. It also requires forming a relationship with a new mentor in the research setting, adding to the stress on the fellow. The postdoctoral programme may interrupt the fellow's academic career path or current clinical practice. The focus of the postdoctoral fellowship is on research and other responsibilities may be temporarily disrupted (Chenitz and Swanson, 1990).

Lev et al (1990) cite Larson and colleagues as noting that less than 0.3% of nurses with doctorates have formal postdoctoral research training. In contrast, all assistant professors hired in the past five years in approximately two-thirds of departments had formal postdoctoral research training (AAU, 2003). A fellow coming from a previous faculty position may, upon starting a fellowship, experience an acute decrease in status as well as a loss of peers. Compared with a faculty position, fellows may find themselves with limitations in support services and office space (Larson et al, 1988 as cited in Lev et al, 1990). Salary is a major issue for nurses considering a postdoctoral fellowship. Stipends for federal traineeships are based on years of professional experience following the award of the doctorate. The stipend ranges from US$35,568 for an individual just out of a doctoral programme to US$51,036 for someone with seven or more years. It is difficult for individuals to consider this level of support when many new assistant professors receive salaries in the high US$50,000 to low US$60,000 range. Some institutions choose to augment these salaries, in the expectation that they will hire the fellow upon completion of the fellowship.

Currently, in nursing, the investment for individuals and institutions in postdoctoral preparation is high, but the payoff is also potentially high. The challenge for the discipline will be to resolve some of the challenges to reap the benefits.

Status of postdoctoral training around the world

An informal survey of educators from several countries revealed that many countries do not have formal postdoctoral training. In some countries, selected institutions provide mentoring to new faculty, or appoint them early to enable them to prepare for the start of the academic year, or provide start-up funds, with the help of national funding agencies such as is done in Korea. Paid sabbatical policies in some countries are granted and some individuals use the year to join international visiting scholar programmes overseas, working with a scholar and conducting research. In the case of other countries, governmental funding is available to the nursing programme for faculty leaves for the same purpose. At the discretion of the nursing school, these awards may be made to new doctoral graduates to hone their research skills or to mid-career faculty to enable them to 're-tool' and update their knowledge and skills.

A pressing problem faced in many countries is the heavy teaching, advisement and service responsibilities allowing little time for research as part of faculty workload. However, nurse leaders around the world are developing an increased appreciation of the ways in which training at this level can enrich nursing science and contribute to the health of the country.

Individually designed international visiting scholar programmes

Budget shortages still remain a significant problem in developing countries like Thailand. The international visiting scholar programme is a financially attractive alternative for scholars from developing countries or other countries where these opportunities are not available, who desire to send an individual to conduct a postdoctoral experience. Typically, the international visiting scholar programme offers two channels for scholars to identify mentoring opportunities. One is personal contact; the individual may directly contact the faculty who has the relevant expertise. The other is by a network approach, the most popular pathway. Scholars can apply through partnerships that their home institution may have with universities in countries such as the USA, Canada and Australia. According to Ketefian (1998), requests for short-term training for international scholars most frequently are requested through government or international agencies, such as the World Health Organization. The host universities not only provide the academic environment, but also facilitate the entry process for the visiting scholars and their families to help them adjust to the new culture. The benefits of the international visiting scholar programme are flexibility, cost savings, and gaining experience in another culture.

International visiting scholar programmes are less time consuming and more flexible than a postdoctoral fellowship. Individuals can enrol in international visiting scholar programmes throughout the year. These experiences also are offered for different periods of time depending on the contact between universities. In addition, these programmes also offer a variety of nursing specialties. Therefore, international visiting scholars can choose the specialty that suits their area of interest.

The cost of the international visiting scholar programmes is lower than the cost of the postdoctoral programme. The international visiting scholars can register in courses to gain additional substantive and methodological expertise.

International visiting scholars gain research and teaching experience. They also may build up the international collaborative network that may include joint research projects and publishing results between universities. The international visiting scholar will bring back images, impressions, and the influences of foreign cultures both on and off the campus. A better understanding of foreign academic systems and cultures is definitely a benefit for the people of both countries.

There is no set system put in place for the international visiting scholar programme due to its flexibility and individualized nature. The scholar may not be able to locate a mentor with the expertise required within the partner university.

Therefore, international visiting scholars may have difficulty in finding universities that offer expertise in their specialty area. Additionally, there are often multiple objectives to be pursued in a short period of time. Thus, international visiting programmes may not result in the same outcomes as in more structured postdoctoral programmes.

The perspective and expectations of the home institution direct and influence the experience for the visiting scholar. In turn, the visiting scholar has the potential to significantly influence the home institution upon return to that setting. International visiting scholars who return to their home countries will have had experiences and formed new visions that will benefit students, faculty members, curriculum development and collaborative research projects. Their experiences will be transmitted through teaching, coaching, consulting and mentoring to students as well as faculty members. International visiting scholars can leverage their experience by assisting in developing the nursing curriculum including the undergraduate, Master's, and PhD programmes at their home institutions.

International visiting scholars can assist in setting up a collaborative research network by continuing to work with their mentors. They can help develop proposals, seek funding and conduct research focusing on cultural differences. Another benefit is in gaining insight into advanced technology, methodology, and research activities. Finally, international visiting scholars will also increase their expertise in their own area of interest. Although these are the expectations for individual international visiting scholar experiences, the culture of the scholar's home institution or country may act as a barrier to achieving the proposed outcomes. For example, a hierarchical system that is strongly embedded in the Eastern world impacts on the infrastructure of academic institutions. Younger faculty are expected to be highly respectful toward senior faculty, regardless of level of education. This situation may limit the progress of young scholars and the ability of the organization to develop younger faculty. This situation poses a challenge to administrators at all levels in the home institutions.

There also are clear benefits for the host institution in having faculty conduct visiting international fellowships. Faculty and students in the host institution gain an appreciation of international nursing scholarship and have the opportunity to build international collegial relationships (Carty et al, 2002). Given the state of technology offered by the Internet and the relative ease of travel, it is now more feasible to develop productive research collaborations. As maintaining and increasing the number of doctorally prepared faculty and established nurse researchers becomes a greater challenge, faculty in the host institution are in turn challenged to mentor their own students while also selectively mentoring international visiting scholars. The result could be a tension between providing research mentorship for students in the host institutions and offering opportunities for a variety of experiences for international visiting scholars. Clearly, the nursing discipline needs to be thoughtful about how to maintain the developing international research collaborations.

Recommendations and implications

Although the benefits of postdoctoral preparation are significant for the individual, future employers and the discipline, doctorally prepared nurses have not sought out postdoctoral training in significant numbers. The shortage of nursing faculty and nurse researchers comes at a critical point for the discipline. Just as the demands for more practitioners, for more faculty, for nursing science and for evidence-based practice have become critical, nursing finds itself struggling to meet these needs. The average age of nurses completing doctoral degrees is significantly higher than for other disciplines (>40 years for nursing, 30 years for doctorates in biomedical and social and behavioural sciences (National Research Council, cited in Sullivan, 2001). Further, the challenges to postdoctoral preparation identified earlier will probably increase in magnitude as the demand for doctorally prepared faculty increases and the opportunities for these nurse scientists without benefit of postdoctoral experience to move to well-paid positions persist.

The nursing discipline cannot afford to ignore the challenges to postdoctoral preparation and must continue efforts to support these experiences for nurse scientists. One approach that is being implemented in a number of institutions is the encouragement of post baccalaureate entry into doctoral study for certain new Bachelor of Science in Nursing graduates. The goal is to create a generation of younger, doctorally prepared scientists who can dedicate time and include a postdoctoral experience in their career trajectory. This matter is discussed elsewhere in this volume. Another tactic is to create mechanisms to supplement the postdoctoral stipends. Countries that do not have formal postdoctoral training opportunities might consider making greater use of the more individualized training available through the international visiting scholar programme offered by some institutions. The continued development of national and international collaborations that foster the exchange of postdoctoral scientists across institutions will contribute to the establishment of a normative expectation for postdoctoral study.

References

Albrecht, M. and Greiner, P. A. (1992). Postdoctoral study: The importance for nursing. *Journal of Nursing Education,* **31**(8), 373–374.

Berlin, L. D., Stennett J. and Bednash, G. D. (2002–2003). *Enrollment and graduations in baccalaureate and graduate programs in nursing.* Washington, DC: American Association of Colleges of Nursing.

Association of American Universities (31 March 1998). *Committee on Postdoctoral Education: Report and Recommendations.* http://www.aau.edu/reports/PostdocRpt.html (accessed on 09.07.2003).

Byrne, M. W. and Keefe, M. R. (2003). A mentored experience (KO1) in maternal-infant research. *Journal of Professional Nursing,* **19**(2), 66–75.

Carty, R., O'Grady, E. T., Wichaikhum, O. A. and Bull, J. (2002). Opportunities in preparing global leaders in nursing. *Journal of Professional Nursing,* **18**(2), 70–77.

Chenitz, W. C. and Swanson, J. M. (1981). The postdoctoral research fellow in nursing: In between the cracks in the academic wall. *Nursing Outlook,* **29**(7), 417–420.

Donaldson, S. K. (2002). Preparation of independent researchers. *Journal of Professional Nursing,* **18**(6), 308–309.

Fisher, A. and Habermann, B. (2001). Transitions: from doctoral preparation to academic career. In: N. L. Chaska (ed.). *The nursing profession: Tomorrow and beyond.* Thousand Oaks, CA: Sage Publications, Inc, pp. 251–261.

Hinshaw, A. S. and Lucas, M. D. (1993). Postdoctoral education – a new tradition for nursing research. *Journal of Professional Nursing,* **9**(6), 309.

International Network for Doctoral Education in Nursing. (2003). *Directory of International Doctoral Programs, 2003.* http://www.umich.edu/~inden/programs/ (accessed on 25.10.2003).

Ketefian, S. (1998). *International training of nurse scholars: Leadership development.* http://www.nursing.umich.edu/oia (accessed 10.10.2003).

Ketefian, S. (1991). Doctoral preparation for faculty roles: Expectations and realities. *Journal of Professional Nursing,* **7**(2), 105–111.

Lev, E., Sourder, E. and Topp, R. (1990). The postdoctoral fellowship experience. *Image: Journal of Nursing Scholarship,* **22**(2), 116–119.

Lowe, A. A., Boyd, M. A. and Brunette, D. M. (1991). Mentoring and pretenure faculty development. *Journal of Dental Education,* **55**, 675–678.

McGivern, D. (2003). The scholars' nursery. *Nursing Outlook,* **51**, 59–64.

McKenna, H. (2000). *The mission and substance of doctoral education in nursing.* International Network for Doctoral Education in Nursing. Available from INDEN website, http://www.umich.edu/~inden/programs/ (accessed on 10.10.2003).

Paul, S. (2000). Postdoctoral training for new doctoral graduates: Taking a step beyond a doctorate. *American Journal of Occupational Therapy,* **55**(2), 227–229.

Singer, M. (2000). Enhancing the postdoctoral experience. *Issues in Science and Technology,* **17**(1), 43–46.

Sullivan, E. J. (2001). The last myth. *Journal of Professional Nursing,* **17**(6), 271–272.

Wood, M. J. (2002). The postdoctoral fellowship. *Clinical Nursing Research,* **11**(2), 123–125.

Chapter 13

Funding for doctoral study and research

Kristen Montgomery

[In our work with international doctoral educators and students, it has become apparent that locating resources to enlarge and enrich doctoral student experiences poses a singular challenge. Thus, we have included a chapter devoted to resources, and we are most grateful to Dr Kristen Montgomery for undertaking this monumental task. *The Editors*]

The websites listed in this chapter represent the best resources available for doctoral students and those considering doctoral study. They also include resources for research. In preparing this chapter every effort was made to include a representative group of resources from the countries that offer nursing doctoral education; however, this was only partially successful. We requested the assistance of colleagues from around the world, and this enabled us to expand the listings included here. We are grateful to all those who provided information for this chapter. In addition to these sites, individuals are encouraged to review the websites of the specific schools that they are interested in attending. Much can be learned from the review of a school's website. For example, one can investigate faculty research interests, faculty funding, if the school's doctoral programme has a specific focus (e.g. women's health or gerontology), the nature of coursework and research experiences, resources and facilities available, other colleges at the university, and the availability of financial aid, research assistantships, student assistantships and courses of interest. The sites listed below include information on obtaining funding for doctoral study and research. They are listed in alphabetical order.

Academy of Finland

http://www.aka.fi

The Academy of Finland is a governmental organization that focuses on research funding and science policy. The goal of the organization is to promote high-level scientific research through long-term quality-based research funding, science and science policy expertise, and efforts to strengthen the position of science and scientific research. Thirteen per cent of total Finnish government revenue supports research at Finnish research universities and research institutes. The Academy of Finland funds research and researcher training.

Ad Astra Chapter of the Association for Women in Science

http://www.ku.edu/~aaawis/gradfund.html

The Ad Astra Chapter of the Association for Women in Science is located in Lawrence, Kansas, USA, and provides scholarships. Scholarships are listed on the web page and are organized by deadline periods (e.g. January–March, April–June, July–September, October–December and ongoing). The website includes a variety of options for doctoral study.

American Association of Colleges of Nursing

http://www.aacn.nche.edu

The American Association of Colleges of Nursing (AACN) is a professional organization that provides information on higher education programmes in nursing in the USA. It is a well-respected organization in the USA that provides a wealth of useful information on all forms of higher education in nursing (e.g. BSN, MSN, ND, DNSc and PhD degrees).

American Association of Colleges of Nursing publication *Indicators of Quality in Research-Focused Doctoral Programs in Nursing* (November 2001)

http://www.aacn.nche.edu/Publications/positions/qualityindicators.htm

The link above provides information from the AACN publication that addresses quality indicators in research-focused doctoral programmes. This resource is particularly useful for those considering doctoral study, so that they can ensure they enter a quality programme that meets their individual goals.

American Association of the History of Nursing – resources

http://www.aahn.org/resource.html

The American Association of the History of Nursing is a professional organization for those interested in nursing history. The organization is based in the USA and includes some research funding opportunities for small pilot projects. Due dates and application guidelines are available through the website.

American Association of University Women

http://www.aauw.org/

The American Association of University Women (AAUW) is a professional organization that supports higher education for women in the USA and internationally. The link above includes information on a variety of fellowships and grants available through the organization. These opportunities are directed towards graduate students and women at other career stages. Information is provided on ordering a fellowship booklet. The AAUW has both a US and an international fellowship programme at the doctoral and postdoctoral levels.

American Cancer Society research programmes and funding

http://www.cancer.org/docroot/RES/RES_O.asp

The American Cancer Society provides information on various funding sources that are supported by the organization. The society only funds proposals that focus on cancer research.

American Nurses Association Ethnic Minority Fellowship Program

http://www.ana.org/emfp/fellowships

The American Nurses Association (ANA) Ethnic Minority Fellowship Program provides funding to qualifying minority students for one to two years. Priority is given to applicants who wish to study psychiatric mental health and substance abuse. The link above includes information on various opportunities that are available including the Clinical Research Post-Doctoral Fellowship, and the Clinical Research Pre-Doctoral Fellowship.

American Nurses Association funding for nursing education

http://www.nursingworld.org/readingroom/edfund.htm

The ANA is the professional nurses association in the USA that represents all nurses. The link provided is one section of the ANA web page that provides information on funding nursing education. The site includes information on the Nurse Reinvestment Act from the Health Resources and Services Administration (HRSA) and how to apply for funds. HRSA is part of the Department of Health and Human Services (DHHS).

ANA's *Online Journal of Issues in Nursing* 'Nursing doctoral education in the Americas'. S. Ketefian, E. Neves and M. Gutiérrez (31 May, 2001)

http://www.nursingworld.org/ojin/topic12/tpc12_8.htm

This is a link to an article on doctoral education in the Americas. The article provides information that may be helpful to those who are considering pursuing doctoral education. See also 'Nursing doctoral education in the United Kingdom and Ireland', in the same journal, by Hugh McKenna and John Cutcliffe.

American Nurses Foundation

http://www.ana.org/anf

The American Nurses Foundation (ANF) offers a variety of grants to support nursing research. Detailed guidelines are available via the website early in the year (January). Some grant opportunities are available to any researcher in any topic area and others specify a particular level of expertise (novice or senior researchers) or area of interest. ANF grants offer small amounts of support that are appropriate for pilot work. Applications are due in early May each year.

American Psychological Association online 1997 doctoral employment survey

http://research.apa.org/des97contents.html

The link above provides general information about graduates of doctoral programmes in the USA. Information includes job types and salary information. The information provided on this site will be useful to those considering applying to doctoral programmes.

Asthma Australia

http://www.asthmaaustralia.org.au/research.html

The Asthma Australia website includes information on the Macquarie Bank Asthma Research Alliance scholarships, which provide funding for PhD research on asthma. An outline of information and applications are available via portable document format (PDF) on the website. The website also includes links to local branches that fund local research, including New South Wales, Queensland, South Australia, Tasmania, Victoria and Western Australia.

Australian College of Midwives, Inc.

http://www.acmi.org.au/

This is the home page for the Australian College of Midwives (ACM). For information on funding opportunities, click on the education section, then go to scholarships. The due date for scholarships through the ACM is 31 March of each year. Funds are available for research projects and are reviewed by a selection committee. A proposal must be submitted to be considered. Funds are also available to attend conferences, for visiting midwives and public education projects.

Australian Department of Health and Ageing

http://www.health.gov.au

The Australian Department of Health and Ageing provides various opportunities for research funding and other projects. Information can be located by clicking on the 'About Us' link and then clicking on 'Tenders and Grants'.

Australian and New Zealand College of Mental Health Nurses

http://www.anzcmhn.org

The above link is to the home page of the Australian and New Zealand College of Mental Health Nurses. Click on the 'Awards and Grants' section to find information on available funding opportunities. A variety of options is available and detailed information is provided on the website.

Australian Research Council Discovery Scheme

http://www.arc.gov.au/grant_programmes/

The link above provides detailed information on the Australian Research Council (ARC) scholarship programmes, deadlines to apply, and priority areas for ARC funding. The web page also includes information on research ethics and national research guidelines.

Australian Rotary Health Research Fund

http://www.rotarnet.com.au/ARHRF/research/research_frameset.htm

The Australian Rotary Health Research Fund supports research in mental health, and administers the Ian Scott Fellowship. Information on the fellowship and general grant support is provided via the web page. Detailed instruction and due dates are listed online. A general fund exists for research aimed at improving the health of Australian citizens.

British Lung Foundation

http://www.britishlungfoundation.com/research.asp

This website provides information on the British Lung Foundation (BLF), the BLF research strategy, goals of the foundation, and grant opportunities.

Detailed information is provided on grant proposal selection criteria. The referees report form, previously funded grants, and application procedures are also included.

BUPA Foundation

http://www.bupafoundation.com

The BUPA Foundation is an independent medical research charity that provides financing for the prevention, relief and cure of sickness and ill health. The Foundation aims to produce long-term benefits that have an impact on the health of both individuals and the whole country. Approximately £1.5 million per year is provided to fund research projects. Research projects in the following areas are supported: clinical excellence, medical research, health at work, epidemiology and communication and care for the elderly.

CAPES (Brazil Government Information)

http://www.capes.gov.br

This website includes information on various scholarships appropriate for doctoral education and research in nursing that are sponsored by the Brazilian government.

Canadian Institute for Health Research Doctoral Research Award

http://www.cihr-iirsc.gc.ca/services/funding/apply/application_packages/training_salary/doc_research_e.shtml

The Canadian Institute of Health Research website includes information on doctoral research awards and the application process. Those interested should apply by 15 October of each year. Detailed information on the award and requirements is provided.

Canadian Nurses Foundation

http://www.canadiannursesfoundation.com/english/welcome.htm

The Canadian Nurses Foundation is a charitable organization promoting health and patient care in Canada. The Foundation provides nursing research grants, study awards for higher education, and financial support for other educational purposes. A key goal of the Foundation is development, dissemination, and implementation of nursing knowledge in Canada. Contact information and general information about the Foundation is provided on the website.

Canadian Society for International Health

http://www.csih.org/opps/fundopps.html

The Canadian Society for International Health website includes information on funding opportunities for Canadians studying for a degree abroad. In addition, the Society provides funding opportunities for research and voluntary work overseas as well as some miscellaneous funding opportunities. The listings on this website are very comprehensive and include detailed contact and application information.

Cancer Research UK

http://www.cancerresearchuk.org

This is a comprehensive website about cancer research that is based in the UK. Click on the 'Science and Research' section for information on funding opportunities, researchers, previously funded grants, institutes and centres and funding management. Annual reports are also available to review on this website under the section titled: 'Funding Committees'. Grant application information is found in the 'Funding and Management' section. A variety of opportunities are available for those interested in cancer research.

Chief Scientist Office (Scotland)

http://www.show.scot.nhs.uk/cso/

The Chief Scientist Office supports and promotes high quality research aimed at improving the sciences offered by the National Health Service of Scotland and the health of the people of Scotland. The website includes information on the revised research strategy, annual reports, the research development scheme, and health-related professions that are included (nursing, midwifery, allied health). A comprehensive list of current research, training, and events opportunities is provided. Application information is available for download.

Churchill Trust – fellowships and scholarships for overseas study

http://www.churchilltrust.com.au/

The Churchill Trust provides scholarships and fellowships to qualifying graduate students who wish to pursue study overseas. Basic information on both scholarships and fellowship opportunities is provided on the website. Detailed application information is also available. The 'frequently asked questions' section is useful for those who are considering an application for one of these awards. Contact information is provided for further information and questions. Information is also provided on previous fellows and their reports.

Clinical Information Access Program (CIAP) professional nursing organizations

http://www.ciap.health.nsw.gov.au/project/cnc/organizations/#aona

This webpage provides a very comprehensive list of scholarship and funding opportunities available in New South Wales, Australia. Brief information about the scholarship or funding source as well as contact information is provided.

Commonwealth Department of Employment, Education, and Youth Affairs (Australia)

http://www.defya.gov.au/esos

The above link provides information on the educational services available for overseas students who are in Australia. General information on programmes, application procedures, frequently asked questions, 'what's new,' and contact information is provided and there are some useful links.

Congress of Aboriginal and Torres Strait Islander Nurses (CATSIN)

http://www.indiginet.com.au/catsin/index.shtml

This organization provides occasional scholarship opportunities for graduate study, provided through the VIERTEL Foundation. The goal of CATSIN is the recruitment and retention of indigenous peoples of Australia in nursing. Contact information and extensive information on CATSIN is provided on the website.

Diabetes Australia Research Trust

http://www.diabetesaustralia.com.au/research/index.html

The Diabetes Australia Research Trust supports diabetes research throughout Australia. Approximately 35 grants are awarded to researchers annually. All proposals are peer reviewed.

Drug and Alcohol Nurses of Australia

http://www.danaonline.org

Drug and Alcohol Nurses of Australia (DANA) is a resource network that provides leadership, professional support and friendship to nurses working with or advocating for people with alcohol and other drug issues and concerned others. The aim of the organization is excellence and ongoing improvement in the quality of nursing care offered to these people. DANA offers a small scholarship of up to AUS$500 to assist in professional development. Applications are accepted anytime. One must be a member of DANA and fill in an application.

Economic and Social Research Council (ESRC)

http://www.esrc.ac.uk/index.asp

The mission of the Economic and Social Research Council (ESRC) is to promote and support high quality basic, strategic and applied research, and related postgraduate training in the social sciences in the UK. The ESRC also strives to advance knowledge and provide trained social scientists. Another function is to provide advice on, and disseminate knowledge, and promote public understanding of the social sciences. Several funding mechanisms are available through the ESRC, including studentships, fellowships, research, research resources and facilities, seminars and workshops, and international opportunities. Detailed information on these options is available from the website.

Endocrine Nurses Society of Australia

http://www.ensa.org.au

The Endocrine Nurses Society of Australia provides a AUS$5000 nursing research grant for endocrine-related proposals. An application must be completed and individuals must meet application criteria to apply. An application form is provided and is due to the Endocrine Nurses Society by 31 July of each year. All information related to the research grant can be found under the section titled 'Research grant'. The site also includes information on scholarships for international travel to an endocrine conference. Individuals may be supported for up to AUS$2500. These funds also require an application due on 31 July of each year.

European Commission

http://www.europa.eu.int

This website provides detailed information on the Sixth Framework Programme for European Research and Technological Development (2002–2006), which may be useful for doctoral students in or from Europe who are deciding on a topic of interest for their dissertation research. The 'Activities' section includes a section titled 'Research and innovation', which also offers information that may be useful to doctoral students and those considering doctoral study. The information on this website is available in several languages.

European Science Foundation

http://www.esf.org

The home page of the European Science Foundation lists several different opportunities for graduate students interested in research funding. There is targeted recruitment of 'young scientists' and programme proposals. The grants page includes information on five different opportunities, private sector sponsorship, and participation of researchers from industry and the private sector in the European Science Foundation activities.

FAFSA: Your Gateway to Financial Aid for Graduate Study

http://gradschool.about.com/library/weekly/aa112502a.htm

This web address is part of the **about.com** network, an organization that provides online information about a variety of topics. Detailed information is provided on obtaining funding for graduate school. This site is not specific to nursing, but offers general information on graduate schools.

Finnish Association of Caring Sciences

http://www.uku.fi/htts/englanti.html

The Finnish Association of Caring Sciences (FACS) is a professional organization that supports and promotes research in nursing science and the application to clinical nursing. FACS also organizes conferences and publishes a journal. Grant opportunities are periodically made available. The address for the board is HTTS, University of Oulu, Department of Nursing and Health Administration, PO Box 5300, FIN 90014, Finland.

Finnish Federation of Nurses

http://www.sairaanhoitajaliitto.fi

Information on this web page is only available in Finnish.

Finnish Foundation of Nursing Education
[In Finnish: Sairaanhoitajien koulutussäätiö]

Address for the Board: SHKS, Erottajankatu 1A 10, 00130 Helsinki, Finland. Currently not available online.

Florence Nightingale Foundation

http://www.florence-nightingale-foundation.org.uk/

The Florence Nightingale Foundation funds a living memorial and strives to advance the study of nursing and the promotion of excellence in nursing practice. Various scholarships are available through the foundation and include funds for travel and research. The web page includes a detailed section on how to apply.

Fogarty International Center

http://www.fic.nih.gov/programs.html

The home page of the Fogarty International Center (FIC) lists several relevant sections including training grants, research grants, and fellowships. The 'International services' section lists the National Institutes of Health (NIH) Visiting Programme for foreign scientists and includes visa and passport information. The mission of FIC is to promote and support scientific research and training internationally to reduce disparities in global health.

Ford Foundation International Fellowships Program

http://www.fordfound.org/news/more/11272000ifp/index.cfm

The Ford Foundation is a resource for innovative people and institutions worldwide that embraces the following goals: strengthen democratic values, reduce poverty and injustice, promote international cooperation and advance human achievement. Detailed information is provided on the Fellowship Program including an introduction, general guidelines, eligibility and the application process.

Fulbright Commissions and Foundations

http://exchanges.state.gov/education/fulbright/commiss.htm

The Fulbright Commissions and Foundations is a group of non-profit organizations that oversee the Fulbright Program abroad. This web page provides application information for US citizens and non-US nationals. Information is also provided on the Fulbright Foreign Scholarship Board and alumni of the programme.

Heart and Stroke Foundation of Canada

http://www.heartandstroke.ca/

The Heart and Stroke Foundation of Canada strives to improve the health of Canadians by preventing and reducing disability and death from heart disease and stroke through research, health promotion and advocacy. The home page of this website includes a list of new opportunities for funding. Individual awards have different criteria and due dates (which are various). An application form, which is also available on the web, must be completed.

Higher Education Funding Council for England *Improving Standards in Postgraduate Research Degree Programmes*

http://www.hefce.ac.uk/pubs/Rdreports/Downloads/report13.htm

The website details findings from a commission to identify indicators that could form the basis of threshold standards in research degree programmes. Information on England, Scotland, and Wales are included. The summary is available online and more detailed sections are available for download. This information may be useful to those considering doctoral study and those who need to decide on a research area for their doctoral research.

International Network for Doctoral Education in Nursing (INDEN)

http://www.umich.edu/~inden/

INDEN is a new professional organization of nurse educators and doctoral students from around the world interested in improving the health of all people through research and doctoral education. The website provides a wealth of information related to doctoral education in nursing and has an international perspective. Useful contact information and doctoral programmes in the USA and worldwide are featured. Information is also provided on conferences that are sponsored by INDEN. INDEN is based at the University of Michigan School of Nursing.

International Transplant Nurses Society

http://www.itns.org

The International Transplant Nurses Society is a worldwide professional nursing organization that represents all areas of transplantation. The goal of the organization is to support clinicians in meeting the ongoing clinical changes and challenges that transplant nurses tackle daily. Research grants in the amount of US$2500 are available and at least two are awarded each year. The website includes a downloadable grant application and information on previous grant recipients.

National Council for Scientific and Technological Development (CNPq in Brazil)

http://www.cnpq.br

This website is available in Portuguese, English and Spanish. The mission of the National Council for Scientific and Technological Development is to promote and stimulate the scientific and technological development of the country and to contribute to the formulation of national science and technology policy. The agency is sponsored by the government and located in Brazil.

National Association of Theatre Nurses

http://www.natn.org.uk/pages/frameawards.html

The National Association of Theatre Nurses (NATN) is a professional organization for nurses who work in the operating room. The web page includes links to several research award opportunities, including: NATN 3M Clinical Fellowship, Regent Medical Award, Johnson & Johnson Medical/Ethicon Nurses Educational Trust, Awards of Merit, The Siobhan Rankin Award, and the Education and Research Fellowship Fund. The goal of the organization is to promote perioperative nursing and to advance nursing practice by encouraging the delivery of clinically effective perioperative care in any setting.

W. K. Kellogg Foundation

http://www.wkkf.org

The mission of the W. K. Kellogg Foundation is to help people help themselves through the practical application of knowledge and resources to improve their quality of life and that of future generations. In the 'News' section of this website one can find information on Community Health Scholars, a postdoctoral programme in community-based participatory care. Applications for this programme are due in early December. Other opportunities are frequently available through the W. K. Kellogg Foundation, so interested individuals should check this website frequently.

Korean Research Foundation

http://www.krf.or.kr

From the home page, one should select either 'English' or 'Korean' to obtain information in the preferred language. The 'Activities' section features a list of various opportunities that are available through the Korean Research Foundation. The foundation offers scholarship programmes for Korean nurses as well as international students studying in Korea.

Korean Science and Engineering Foundation

http://www.kosef.re.kr/global

The Korean Science and Engineering Foundation works to enhance the research capability for a prosperous future. The home page includes links to several research and funding opportunities, some of which may be useful for doctoral students in nursing. The 'Program' section lists some additional information.

Medical Research Council of South Africa

http://www.mrc.ac.za

The goal of the Medical Research Council of South Africa is building a healthy nation through research. The 'Funding opportunities' section lists several opportunities that are currently available through the Medical Research Council of South Africa. Some funding is also available for travel grants.

Medical Research Council of the UK

http://www.mrc.ac.uk

The Medical Research Council (MRC) of the UK is a similar organization that is relevant to research in the UK. The 'Call for proposals' section includes information on several listings for various research grants. The 'Studentships' section includes information on applying for a studentship and specific priority areas. The mission of the MRC is to promote research in all areas of medical and related science with the aims of improving the health and quality of life in the UK. The MRC is taxpayer-funded. More information on funding can be obtained from the 'Funding' page of the website.

Michigan State University Library's grants for individuals list – Nursing

http://www.lib.msu.edu/harris23/grants/3nursing.htm

The Michigan State University is a public, state-supported institution of higher learning. The web page includes a list of Michigan-based and more broad resources that are relevant to nursing. Links are provided to specific guidelines and brief information is included about the award or scholarship.

Ministry of Education – Thailand

http://www.moe.go.th/read46

This website provides information on opportunities that may be of interest to nurses pursuing their doctoral degree. The Content on this website is in Thai. Graduate student support is available, although in most cases this is accessed through the university after the student has enrolled.

National Health and Medical Research Council Schemes (Australia)

http://www.health.gov.au/nhmrc/

The National Health and Medical Research Council (NHMRC) schemes function to consolidate many research activities, including government, healthcare providers, teaching and research institutions, public and private corporations, and consumers. The NHMRC also functions to raise the standard of individual and public health throughout Australia, to foster development of consistent health standards between various states and health territories, and to foster medical research and training, including ethics. The website provides information on palliative care graduate scholarships and extensive information on research review procedures. The 'Scholarships' section includes a link to an A–Z guide of multiple options for scholarships and research funding. Information is available for download via Portable Document Format (PDF).

National Heart Foundation postgraduate scholarships (non-medical) and fellowships tenable in Australia and overseas

http://www.heartfoundation.com.au

Cardiovascular disease is the leading cause of death in Australia. The National Heart Foundation (NHF) was established in 1958 to pursue new knowledge about the heart and its diseases and to disseminate that knowledge. The NHF funds research into the causes, prevention, treatment and diagnosis of cardiovascular disease and related disorders. The NHF invests about AUS$6 million into these programmes each year. The section on 'Program objectives' provides detailed information on specific fellowships, scholarships and grants for aid and travel.

National Institute of Nursing Research

http://www.nih.gov/ninr

The National Institute of Nursing Research (NINR) is the funding source for nursing research at the national level in the USA. NINR is one of the institutes within the National Institutes of Health, the main funding agency of the US government for biomedical research. It offers several options for doctoral and postdoctoral funding for US citizens, both for study/training as well as for nursing research.

National League for Nursing

http://www.nln.org

The National League for Nursing (NLN) provides funding for nursing education research based on priorities established by the organization. Proposals for funding are due each year in early March. In addition, through the Foundation for Nursing Education, the NLN administers scholarships for nurses pursuing graduate degrees with a focus on teaching.

National Multiple Sclerosis Society of Australia

http://www.msaustralia.org.au/research/how_to_apply_for_funding.htm

The National Multiple Sclerosis Society of Australia offers project grants, postdoctoral fellowships, postgraduate research scholarships, seed grants and summer vacation scholarships. Detailed information on each of these options is provided on the website. Research/experiences must focus on multiple sclerosis.

National Nursing Centers Consortium – Americans for Nursing Shortage Relief

http://www.nationalnursingcenters.com/NNCC_Partners/partners_Americans_For_Nursing_Shortage_Relief.htm

The purpose of the National Nursing Centers Consortium – Americans for Nursing Shortage Relief is to assure quality healthcare in the USA by supporting nurse education and training and by building an adequate supply of nurses.

National Research Foundation – South Africa

http://www.nrf.ac.za

The National Research Foundation of South Africa funds research relevant to the people of South Africa. The 'Funding' section lists multiple funding options and detailed guidelines for each. The 'Student' section lists two options for support: (i) free-standing bursaries, scholarships and fellowships, and (ii) grant holder-linked assistantships and bursaries. The website includes an informational guide to student support. The home page features additional useful information including databases, publications, discussion groups, events, rated researchers and links.

National Science Foundation

http://www.nsf.gov

The mission of the National Science Foundation is to promote the progress of science; to advance national health, prosperity, and welfare; to secure the national defence; and other purposes. A variety of grant opportunities are available in the broad programme areas of biology, computer and information sciences, cross-cutting programmes, education, engineering, geosciences, international, math, physical sciences, polar, science statistics, and social and behavioural sciences. Detailed information on application procedures and requirements is available via the website.

New South Wales Health Professional Nursing Groups

http://www.health.nsw.gov.au/nursing/pros.html

The New South Wales Health Professional Nursing Groups offer several scholarship opportunities for nurses. The link provides information on the 12 different scholarships with contact information and brief criteria for application.

New South Wales Nurses' Association

http://www.nswnurses.asn.au

The New South Wales Nurses' Association is the professional organization for nurses living in New South Wales, Australia. Several scholarship opportunities are available, including the E. C. Trust Scholarship, the Lions Nurses' Scholarships, and the New South Wales Scholarships. The E. C. Trust Scholarship application is due on 31 July of each year. The Lions Nurses' Scholarships category A and B are due on 30 November of each year. The New South Wales Nursing Scholarship Fund offers financial support for postgraduate study for registered nurses employed in the New South Wales public health system who undertake study at a New South Wales or other approved university.

Nurses Educational Funds

http://www.n-e-f.org

Nurses Educational Funds is a not-for-profit organization that provides funding for graduate education for BSN-prepared nurses who are US citizens. Funding decisions are made by a board. Application process and criteria are available via the website.

Nurses' Registration Board of New South Wales, Research and Development Scholarships – Category 5

http://www.nursesreg.health.nsw.gov.au

On the home page, click on 'Scholarships for nurses' to find information on funding opportunities. Funds through the Nurses' Registration Board of New South Wales are available for education, research and attendance at meetings.

Nursing Outlook Online, Knowledge development in nursing: our historical roots and future opportunities. S. R. Gortner (March/April 2000)

http://www.nursing.niu.edu/lash/N513/Gortner%20article.htm

The link is to a full text article that discusses knowledge development in nursing from a historical perspective. Susan Gortner is a leading nurse expert in this area and *Nursing Outlook* is a respected publication. The article provides information that will likely be useful for nurses pursuing doctoral education in nursing.

Peterson's Grants for Graduate and Post-Doctoral Study

Available at Amazon.com

Peterson's guide is a most useful resource to learn about grants that are available for graduate and postdoctoral study. This book is available for purchase online from Amazon.com or in other bookstores. It is a general reference guide and is not specific to nursing, but may be useful for nurses who are pursuing advanced education.

Queensland Cancer Foundation

http://www.qldcancer.com.au/

The Queensland Cancer Foundation provides funding to various cancer-related projects. On the home page, click on 'research' to find more information on the various opportunities. The overall aim of the organization is to reduce the impact of cancer – particularly the suffering it causes – and ultimately to eliminate the disease by raising funds to improve care through research. Thus, proposals submitted for funding to the Queensland Cancer Foundation should address this aim in some way.

Queensland Nursing Council

http://www.qnc.qld.gov.au/

The Queensland Nursing Council offers several research grants and scholarships to nurses practising in Queensland, Australia. The organization was founded in 1993 to regulate nursing practice in Queensland.

Re-envisioning the PhD Project

http://www.grad.washington.edu/envision

This project was started to provide a forum for all stakeholders in doctoral education for dialogue on the future of the PhD degree, and to take a fresh look at the degree with the goal of revitalizing it. It is interdisciplinary in nature; while it began as a dialogue within the USA, it has expanded to include other countries as well. For more information on this project see Chapter 4.

Rockefeller Foundation

http://www.rockfound.org

The Rockefeller Foundation describes its mission as furthering the wellbeing of mankind throughout the world. It is a knowledge-based global foundation with a commitment to enrich and sustain the lives and livelihoods of poor and excluded people throughout the world. The home page lists several fellowship opportunities. The section labelled 'Programs' details the different 'themes' that the foundation is interested in. These include creativity and culture, food security, health equality and working communities. The 'Information for applicants' section provides detailed information on application procedures and the long-term goals of the foundation, which should be the focus of the application.

Royal College of Nursing Australia

http://www.rcna.org.au

The Royal College of Nursing Australia is the professional organization for all nurses of Australia. Several scholarship opportunities are available. Detailed application instructions are provided on the website.

Royal College of Nursing Research and Development Co-ordinating Centre – research funding

http://www.man.ac.uk/rcn/ukwide/ukrfund.html

The Royal College of Nursing (RCN) is the professional nursing organization in the UK. The RCN Research and Development Co-ordinating Centre oversees the research operations of the RCN. The link above goes directly to a comprehensive list of UK funding sources for research and scholarships. Where available, information is provided on requirements, due date, and any other relevant information needed to apply. The Research and Development Co-ordinating Centre also provides numerous other resources to facilitate research in the UK and internationally.

Scholarships for study and research in the USA

http://www.ghi-dc.org/guide10/frameus.html

The above web address links to a very comprehensive international list of funding sources for study in the USA. Requirements for the awards and due dates are provided when available.

Scottish Executive Fellowships for Nursing

http://www.nmpdu.org/fellowships

The Scottish Executive Fellowships for Nursing were first introduced in 1999 by the Minister of Health and Community Care to encourage nurses, midwives, health visitors and multidisciplinary teams to develop innovative ideas to improve patient care in the National Health Service of Scotland. Awards may be used for travel, education or practice development. The panel considers proposals in the following areas: supporting vulnerable people, health of children, women-centred maternity services, interventions with acutely ill patients, mental health and wellbeing, support of patients with chronic diseases, involving families in care, clinical leadership, clinical decision making, innovative use of technology in care delivery, and multidisciplinary/multi-agency approach to care. Fellowships are awarded annually.

Sigma Theta Tau, International

http://www.nursingsociety.org

Sigma Theta Tau, International (STTI) is the worldwide honour society for nurses. STTI offers various research resources that may be useful to doctoral students in nursing. In addition, STTI also offers funding for small pilot studies. These opportunities have various due dates and requirements, which may be obtained from the website.

Society for Medical Anthropology

http://www.medanthro.net/funding/postdoc

The Society for Medical Anthropology is a professional organization for anthropologists specializing in medical anthropology. The website includes a list of research funding links, some of which are relevant to nursing research. Detailed information can be obtained via the links.

Social Sciences and Humanities Research Council of Canada

http://www.sshrc.ca/web/home_e.asp

The Social Sciences and Humanities Research Council of Canada provides various funding mechanisms for research. To find more information on the website, click on 'Apply for funding.' Information is included on programmes for graduate students, postdoctoral researchers, faculty, community and non-profit organizations, post-secondary institutions, and scholarly associations. Each of these opportunities has different criteria and due dates. These can be found on the web page for those who are interested in additional information.

State of São Paulo Research Foundation

http://www.fapesp.br

The information on this website is available in Portuguese, English and Spanish. The home page features multiple scholarship opportunities, including at the Master's, doctoral, and postdoctoral levels. Detailed instructions are provided for these awards. This organization is one of the main agencies in Brazil to foster scientific and technological research in the country.

The 2000 National Doctoral Programme Survey (released 17 October, 2001)

http://survey.nagps.org/index.php

This web page provides the results of a survey on doctoral education practices and characteristics of doctoral graduates that was conducted by the National Association of Graduate and Professional Students, USA. The organization was founded in 1986 and has provided doctoral students with relevant data since its inception. For the survey that is linked here, there were over 32,000 respondents. Specific sections of the results are divided into categories of interest, including recent PhDs. One can view results, discuss the survey online with others, and learn about the survey methodology. This project was funded by the Alfred P. Sloan Foundation.

Transcultural Nursing Society's list of scholarships and financial aid

http://www.tcns.org/menu/menu36.shtml

The Transcultural Nursing Society is a professional organization for nurses who are interested in culturally competent nursing care. The organization offers a certification programme through which one can become a certified transcultural nurse. The website features a resource page that includes information on scholarships from a variety of sources. The list is very comprehensive.

UK Department of Health Research Governance Framework (United Kingdom)

http://www.doh.gov.uk/research/rd3/nhsranddd/researchgovernance.htm

This web page includes information for England, Scotland, Wales, and Northern Ireland; it provides governmental links related to research. The website includes information on research priority areas, calls for proposals and other funding sources.

University of Michigan Horace H. Rackham Graduate School fellowships

http://www.rackham.umich.edu/Fellowships/rackhamf.html

The University of Michigan is a state-assisted institution of higher learning in the USA. This web link includes a variety of international fellowships for doctoral education. Some are local, but there are many that are available to international students.

Writing Your Dissertation: Invisible Rules for Success (R. S. Brause)

Available at Amazon.com

Writing Your Dissertation: Invisible Rules for Success is a useful book that provides general information on completing the dissertation process. The book is easy to read.

Subject Index

Notes
In order to save space in the index the following abbreviations have been used:
AACN – American Association of Colleges of Nursing
CAPES – Foundation Coordination for the Improvement of Higher Education
INDEN – International Network for Doctoral Education in Nursing
PFF – Preparing Future Faculty Programme